dispel depression

the complete easy-to-follow diet and activity plan

carolyn humphries
with charlotte glazzard

foulsham

LONDON • NEW YORK • TORONTO • SYDNEY

foulsham

The Publishing House, Bennetts Close, Cippenham, Slough,
Berkshire, SL1 5AP, England

Foulsham books can be found in all good bookshops and direct from
www.foulsham.com

ISBN-13: 978-0-572-03219-7
ISBN-10: 0-572-03219-6

Cover top right photograph © Anthony Blake Photograph Library
Cover bottom left photograph © Superstock
Illustrations by Ruth Murray © W. Foulsham & Co. Ltd

A CIP record for this book is available from the British Library

The Copyright Act prohibits (subject to certain very limited
exceptions) the making of copies of any copyright work or of
a substantial part of such a work, including the making of
copies by photocopying or similar process. Written
permission to make a copy or copies must therefore
normally be obtained from the publisher in advance. It is
advisable also to consult the publisher if in any doubt as to
the legality of any copying which is to be undertaken.

Neither the editors of W. Foulsham & Co. Ltd nor the
author nor the publisher take responsibility for any possible
consequences from any treatment, procedure, test, exercise,
action or application of medication or preparation by any
person reading or following the information in this book.
The publication of this book does not constitute the practice
of medicine, and this book does not attempt to replace any
diet or instructions from your doctor. The author and
publisher advise the reader to check with a doctor before
administering any medication or undertaking any course of
treatment or exercise.

Printed in Great Britain by Creative Print and Design (Wales), Ebbw Vale

Contents

Introduction

D epression is something that affects an increasing number of people. Fortunately, it is now recognised as an illness and something we can take action to combat. Obviously, the severity of depression suffered by individual people varies enormously, and this book in no way suggests that serious illness can be cured by food and activity alone. However, a carefully controlled diet and activity plan can – and will – help sufferers of mild depression to lift themselves out of their depression and back to normal. It can also support courses of conventional and complementary medicines and treatments being followed by those with a more severe problem, helping them to maintain their health and hasten their return to full strength.

We all have 'off days' but if you've been feeling down for more than a couple of weeks, lack energy and your usual ability to make decisions, and you can't seem to 'snap out of it', the chances are you are suffering from a form of depression. There may be an obvious reason why you are feeling down – a traumatic event, the death of someone close to you, a divorce – or you may have no idea why you are so low. Either way, if you have a depressive disorder, it can affect every aspect of your life: how you eat and sleep, your outlook, your self-esteem, even your physical appearance. It won't just go away either. So ignore people who tell you to 'pull yourself together'. You are probably desperately trying to do just that, but to no avail.

The first thing to do is to go to your doctor who will assess if you are clinically depressed. There are many types of depression, of varying intensity. You may need treatment, either in the form of medication or therapy. I shall explain more about the different types on page 11.

If you are just going through a 'blue' period or have a mild form of depressive disorder, following the advice in this book will help put you back in control of your world. If you have moderate depression and are perhaps on prescribed medication, there is still lots of information here to help you get through this period in your life. Keep in mind, though, that you should go back to the doctor if your symptoms persist.

However, if you are diagnosed with severe depression, in whatever form, you will need to focus on your medical treatment before you start thinking about the recommendations in this book. But as soon as you do feel ready, you will find that the ideas and suggestions will be a help and support to your conventional treatment.

The first thing I shall concentrate on is your diet. When you are depressed, a nutritious, balanced diet is what you most need but, ironically, it is most likely that you either can't face eating at all or you go on binges, craving unhealthy sweet, sugary and fatty foods. Consequently, you are likely to end up suffering from various deficiencies of important nutrients, which can affect your brain's chemistry and make you feel even worse. The diet plans I have put together will help you to avoid this and will actually boost your sense of wellbeing, helping you to dispel those feelings of negativity.

Physical activity is also vital. I have teamed up with Charlotte Glazzard, BSc (Hons) Sports Science, a personal trainer who is currently studying for an MSc in physiotherapy. She explains why you need to exercise, as well as eat and sleep well, and has designed the perfect programme that's easy to follow – and to stick to. That doesn't mean a punishing exercise regime that sets you up to fail, but sensible, simple exercises to help you feel better. This programme, coupled with a no-effort eating regime, plus everything else you need to get through each day positively, will gradually build your confidence and physical wellbeing.

The programme is designed for sufferers of depression. However, it may also assist those of you who are supporting someone with depression, by providing detailed guidance as to how best you can help them towards recovery.

There are no instant fixes here. It will take time, so be patient. But rest assured that all you have to do is follow the plans laid out for you – all the thinking has been done for you. Hopefully, with the help of this book, you are just a few chapters – or weeks – away from a much brighter future.

chapter one

Finding out about Depression

irst, let's look more closely at depression, its causes and how to recognise whether you are affected. One important thing to remember is that having depression is not a sign of weakness. It is an illness that can be treated.

The symptoms

Okay, so you've been feeling down a lot lately; but do you have depression? The range of symptoms is wide and they manifest in a variety of ways. You may not experience all of them and, individually, they do not necessarily mean you have a depressive disorder. Many of these symptoms can be caused by a whole variety of physical illnesses too. That is why, if you suffer two or more of these symptoms regularly, it is very important that you see your doctor to diagnose your problem accurately.

The symptoms to be aware of are:

- Persistent feelings of sadness, emptiness or anxiousness
- Insomnia
- Inability to wake up and face the day
- Permanent feelings of fatigue and lack of energy
- Lack of concentration and inability to remember things or make decisions
- Irritability and restlessness
- Lack of self-esteem

- Guilty feelings
- Loss of appetite and/or weight
- Weight gain and massive comfort-eating
- Physical illnesses with no apparent cause, such as persistent headache, general aches and pains, upset tummy
- Lack of interest in hobbies and leisure
- Loss of sexual appetite
- Suicidal tendencies.

What causes depression?

One in 10 people will suffer some form of depression at some time during their life. Most frequently, a particular incident can start the ball rolling, such as a chronic illness, a bereavement, a broken relationship, serious financial problems or a dramatic downward change to your lifestyle. Any of these, particularly if combined with stress, can initiate an attack.

Some forms of depression are hereditary. However, this does not mean that if you have a depressive parent you will automatically suffer from depression yourself.

Who is most at risk?

Anybody can suffer from depression, from the average man in the street to the rich and famous. For some reason, however, women are more likely to be affected than men and some specific groups of people are more susceptible than others, including:

- Those who have a family history of depression
- Those from severely underprivileged backgrounds
- Those who have suffered sexual, physical or mental abuse
- Those unable to cope adequately with their day-to-day life (this is called a maladaptive coping mechanism).

Different types of depression

Any form of depressive disorder will make you feel sad, worthless, exhausted and unable to function normally. However, these negative thoughts are not permanent: they are part of the illness and will gradually disappear as you recover.

There are quite a few types of depression, of different intensities, which will need varying degrees of treatment. It is important to recognise how extensive the symptoms are and how different the problems can be.

Clinical depression

This is simply a term that means the depression is severe enough to need some form of medical treatment.

Dysthymia or chronic depression

This can be quite mild but there is a continuous, long-term feeling of sadness and inability to function efficiently.

Unipolar depression (also known as major depression)

Major depression is more disabling. The patient will feel moody and sad and will also find they are unable to eat, sleep or work properly and are incapable of having a good time. This may occur in bouts.

Double depression

This is a combination of dysthymia with bouts of major depression (see above).

Bipolar disorder (also known as manic depression)

Manic depression is a severe and difficult illness. It manifests itself in mood swings, varying from deep depression to elation or mania. The changes are usually gradual but on occasion can be quite dramatic. When in the depressive cycle, the patient may experience any or all of the symptoms of chronic depression (see above). When in the manic cycle, they may behave inappropriately in public or have feelings of elation or irritability. They may also suffer from a further range of symptoms, including insomnia; hyperactivity; lack of concentration; irrational judgement; delusional behaviour; erratic, fast or loud speech; heightened sexual appetite.

People who develop this disorder at a relatively young age and go undiagnosed are more likely to also abuse alcohol and/or other substances, which will make their condition worse. They are also more likely to develop other serious mental disorders requiring medical treatment, such as anorexia, bulimia, attention deficit hyperactivity disorder (ADHD) or panic attacks.

Psychotic depression

This is a severe form of major depression. Symptoms of this illness include deep agitation and anxiety, hallucinations (both seen and heard), delusional thinking and the inability to judge actions rationally. Medical help must be sought urgently, as the patient will be in serious danger.

Atypical depression

Atypical depression is very common in adolescent girls. It ebbs and flows, with the sufferer experiencing 'high' moods when in company, plummeting to profound 'lows' when alone. The classic symptoms are oversleeping and an inability to get out of bed in the mornings; overeating; panic attacks; over-sensitivity to and a history of romantic rejection; a leaden feeling in the arms and legs. Chocolate is usually the favourite comfort food. If undiagnosed, it can continue for life.

Postnatal depression

There are actually three types of postnatal depression.

Baby blues: This condition is very common and is suffered to a greater or lesser extent by 60 to 80 per cent of new mothers. The symptoms usually appear a few days after the birth of the baby. The mother may experience sudden mood swings, ranging from desperately sad to positively elated. She may become very tearful for no reason, as well as irritable, impatient and anxious. This usually lasts only a few days, or a couple of weeks at most, and is mainly caused by hormonal imbalances in the body following the birth. A healthy diet, plus the support of family and friends and her health visitor is usually all that is needed to overcome it. It is important that she does remember to do the recommended postnatal exercises. Please note that the exercises in this book are not suitable for a very new mother, but may be started as soon as she has been declared fit at her postnatal check (speak to a health visitor or doctor first).

Postpartum depression: This can happen after a few days or even after a few months following childbirth. The symptoms are similar to baby blues but do not clear up. If after a few days the new mother still cannot function properly and feels unable to cope on a day-to-day basis, perhaps even having panic attacks, she needs help. She should see a doctor or health visitor as soon as possible. A nutritious diet and plenty of rest are absolute essentials, and she may also need counselling or medication.

Postpartum psychosis: This is a rare but very serious condition, which usually starts within three months of the birth. The first symptoms are severe insomnia, agitation and anger. Sufferers may have hallucinations, become deluded and out of touch with reality. In severe cases, they may even feel suicidal. Urgent medical intervention is vital to safeguard the wellbeing of both mother and baby.

Premenstrual dysphoric disorder

This is a severe form of premenstrual tension (PMT) and affects fewer than five per cent of women. It has similar symptoms to PMT but involves much more pronounced depression, mood swings and irritability. It can occur up to two weeks before menstruating and throughout the period of bleeding – which doesn't leave a lot of respite between cycles! It is important that the sufferer seeks help.

Seasonal affective disorder (SAD)

This occurs in people who are particularly sensitive to the reduction in daylight during the winter months. People affected can feel sad, irritable and moody with little or no energy. They oversleep and overeat. Once spring arrives, they become revitalised and happy again. There is no cure, but diet and exercise can help.

Dealing with negativity

The miserable feelings you get when you suffer from depression are very real. They are caused by chemical changes in the brain.

When you are functioning normally, your brain operates as a finely tuned control centre, telling your body to do everything from thinking to eating and sleeping. It sends messages to, and receives them from, the rest of your body via chemicals called neurotransmitters in the nerve cells. The levels of these neurotransmitters determine, amongst other things, your emotional wellbeing. If too few are transmitted, you will feel depressed and negative. If the level is raised, you will feel happy and elated.

When you experience a depression-inducing situation – like divorce, bereavement or chronic illness, for example – the resulting stress causes your brain to reduce the production of neurotransmitters, so causing the desperate feelings.

That's where anti-depressants, therapy, diet and exercise can all help. Each of them, individually or in combination, can raise the quantity of neurotransmitters in your body and so help counteract the negative emotions. Obviously, if your depression is quite severe or prolonged, you may need medication and therapy to help get you back on track. For milder conditions, diet, exercise and an organised, simple lifestyle may be sufficient.

chapter two

How to Help Someone with Depression

I t can be difficult to know what to do if you think a relative or friend is depressed. It is common for the depressed person to be the last one to realise they are actually suffering from an illness. Usually the symptoms creep up gradually and the sufferer just feels they are not getting on with things as well as they normally do, and that they are being weak-willed. It doesn't occur to them that they might actually be ill.

By far the best thing to do is to try to get them to talk about it. Sometimes just having someone else listen to their problems is enough to help them to put things in perspective and feel better. So let them talk – and talk, and talk – if that's what they want to do. If you suspect things are more serious, you may need to do the talking, but do remember the following:

- If you believe they might be clinically depressed, then gently and sensitively raise the issue. They may not want to discuss it, but encourage them to as best you can. Be gentle, not bullying.

- Suggest that they should see their GP and reassure them that the doctor will be able to help whatever the problem. It may be helpful if you offer to go with them. If they get angry or upset, do not push the issue.

- Always offer encouragement, not criticism. If they are having trouble doing normal everyday things – like getting out of bed or getting dressed properly – just gently encourage them to try.

- Don't ever tell them to 'pull themselves together'.

- If they are feeling hopeless or useless, reassure them that it's not their fault. Remind them that they may be ill but that, with help, they will get better.

- The longer the problem continues, the more necessary it becomes for you to persuade them to see their doctor.

Understanding the problems

It is important to note that the word 'depressed' is often used very loosely and inaccurately and this does give us a wrong perspective on what depression really is. Depression is an illness caused by chemical imbalances in the brain. It is not the same as when you are just feeling down. Understanding the effects of real depression is important if you are trying to help someone who is suffering from it. Here are a few facts to bear in mind.

- A depressed person does not have the same control over their feelings that most people do. This is why medication can be important because it restores the chemical imbalance enough to help them regain control and deal with life issues in a more normal way.

- They find even the simplest of everyday tasks difficult – this is where you can be a real help.

- They are likely to go over and over the same ground in their minds. Allowing them to talk it out can help to resolve that process, so listening is a valuable skill.

- You need to allow them time to reach their own conclusions. The answer to one or more issues may be obvious to you. You can make constructive suggestions but they have to find their own solutions. When they do, resist the temptation to remind them you told them that some time ago.

- They need to know that you're there to listen and to help with practical things as well as emotional matters. Keep reassuring them.

- They need a good diet – but they probably can't summon the energy to prepare proper meals. If you can help on a day-to-day basis, try to make sure they follow one of the eating plans in this book – either the snack one starting on page 39 or the three-meals-a-day one on pages 68–95. If you are preparing meals for them, you don't have to follow the plan. Just make sure they get plenty of the nutrients listed in How Foods Can Help (see page 24). If you are following the plan, remember that the added fruit, vegetables, whole grains, nuts and seeds are the vital extras that help their mental state. Note that, much as it goes against the grain, I have deliberately chosen lots of convenience foods – but with healthy additions – so that people with depression who are looking after themselves have hardly any preparation to do. You could, of course, substitute home-cooked foods for the ready meals suggested (and it will be all to the good if you do!).

- They may need help to plan their day. If you are not living with them, try to telephone them every morning and go through this. Don't be too assertive or expect too much, but do help them to focus on a few simple tasks they can aim to achieve during the course of the day.

- They may come up with excuses for not doing things. If this happens, be firm but not dismissive, and help them to reason away their fears.

- They may try to resort to excess alcohol or other non-prescribed drugs to try to relieve their misery. This is easier to control if you live with them. But if not, try to remind them quietly that it will just make matters worse. Of course, there is no harm in having a small drink before a meal to stimulate the appetite or a glass of wine with a meal if that makes life more pleasurable but that is very different from turning to the bottle for solace. If you suspect they are becoming dependant on alcohol or other drugs, you **must** try to get them to seek help.

- It can be a great relief to them to have decisions taken for them. So occasionally – if you feel it is appropriate – you may wish to try to do this, perhaps by encouraging them to get out and about. You could, for example, call at lunchtime and tell them to have their supper early so that you can pick them up at six and take them to the cinema. This will give them something to focus on to help them think constructively.

- They need regular company. Try to arrange this or, if that is difficult, try to get friends or family to telephone or even text them. Being alone for long periods can be difficult to deal with and will only give them opportunities for dwelling on their problems.

- They often find it difficult to make any kind of physical effort. To make sure they follow their exercise routine, offer to come round and do it with them.

- You should never ignore any talk of suicide or wanting to harm themselves. It could be serious, so you must make them see a doctor immediately. You won't make them more likely to do something by insisting they talk to a professional.

You have feelings too!

Helping someone who is depressed is not easy and can take its toll on the carer. Don't forget your own needs as well as theirs. There may be times when you feel your impatience and frustration rising, when you want to take them by the shoulders and shout, 'For heaven's sake, just get on with it!' – or you want to burst into tears yourself because you feel you are just not able to help them.

Give yourself regular breaks – have a bath, go for a walk, talk to someone else about yourself, not them – to help you re-charge your own batteries. If the person's depression has been going on long enough without improvement to raise this reaction in you, it is likely that they should go back to their doctor for more advice on how to improve matters. In most cases, the doctor will have expected the patient gradually to get better and will have alternative treatment options open to them if this is not happening.

chapter three

The First Steps to Recovery

I f you are reading this book, you are already taking your first steps on the road to recovery. But before you start on the diet and exercise plans, it is essential that you make an appointment to see your medical practitioner, if you have not already done so, in order to obtain a proper diagnosis of your condition.

Talk to your doctor

Your doctor will give you a thorough examination to rule out other illnesses and ask you a range of questions about your symptoms and your history. You need to try to be as open as possible, mentioning everything, however trivial it may seem. Your doctor will also check that the symptoms are not the effects of taking other prescribed drugs, of drug or alcohol abuse, or of another medical condition such as hypothyroidism or diabetes.

If you are diagnosed as clinically depressed, your doctor may prescribe anti-depressants or, if appropriate, refer you to a psychiatrist who may prescribe medication, electro-convulsive therapy (ECT) and/or psychotherapy. Don't panic at the idea of ECT – it's is nothing like you would imagine from the movies. It is a highly sophisticated, very effective treatment for severe depression, and is given under an anaesthetic, so the patient knows nothing about it. Psychotherapy is nothing to fear, either; it comes in different forms, all of which can have enormous benefits.

If you have other problems related to your depression, such as alcoholism, drug abuse or eating or anxiety disorders, your doctor will deal with treatment for these at the same time.

Will I become addicted to anti-depressants?

You may well be reluctant to visit your doctor because you have heard that they are likely to prescribe anti-depressants, which can be addictive. This is a perfectly reasonable apprehension and one you should discuss with your doctor. It is important to remember that medication does not provide a cure in itself, but it can be an excellent way to re-balance the chemicals in your brain that are causing you to feel the way you do. You can then relax and get on with your day-to-day life, while you resolve the issues that have caused the problem. You will be under the doctor's supervision all the time, and they will help you to find ways to improve your health. If you had sprained your ankle, you would not refuse to take painkillers: this is no different.

Herbs, herbal remedies and supplements

Many people feel uncomfortable about taking medication and prefer the idea of natural, alternative therapies rather than conventional medicines. These have been found to be very effective for some people and, indeed, some doctors recommend them. Natural herbal remedies in particular have become very popular in recent years and are now widely available over the counter in pharmacists and health shops.

It is important to note, however, that 'natural' does not necessarily mean 'safe' and some herbal remedies are extremely strong. Only certain forms may be taken by mouth and many need to be diluted before application. For this reason, you should consult a qualified herbalist before taking any herbal remedy and always follow any instructions on the packet extremely carefully. You should also inform your doctor if you are considering taking herbal remedies, as some herbs will interfere with conventional medication and treatment.

There are, of course, many commercial products on the market that contain herbs – such as bath and shower foams, soaps, candles, herb-filled pillows, and so on – all of which can create a relaxed atmosphere and make you feel pampered, whilst also helping you to sleep. These are perfectly safe for most people and are an excellent way of indulging yourself when you feel you need a treat.

Herbs that may help

Basil, camomile, clary sage, lavender, lemonbalm, Jamaica dogwood, wild lettuce, skullcap, fir needle, yarrow, neroli, orange, rose, sandalwood, ylang ylang, valerian, passionflower, Californian poppy, peppermint and fennel are all good for promoting calm and sleep.

Bergamot, camomile, clary sage, frankincense, geranium, grapefruit, jasmine, lavender, lemongrass, melissa, neroli, orange, patchouli, rose, sandalwood, Spanish sage, and ylang ylang are said to help to alleviate feelings of depression. Marjoram should be avoided, however.

Some of the above may be taken as dietary supplements or brewed in hot water to make a soothing drink. Others should be added to your bath water or used in oil form in an essence burner. Again, you should check labels carefully to make sure that you are using them in the correct way.

Always check with your doctor or a qualified herbalist before taking any herbal remedy, and always follow the instructions for dosage and application.

The following are available as dietary supplements, to be taken by mouth.

S-Adenosyl Methionine (SAMe): This is a naturally occurring compound found in all human beings. It helps your brain to produce neurotransmitters and so assists in developing a positive mental attitude.

5-Hydroxitryptophan (5-HTP): This is an amino acid that helps your brain to produce serotonin, so boosting your mental and emotional wellbeing.

Ginkgo biloba: This herb increases the blood flow to the brain, thus stimulating it, and is thought to have a positive effect on your mood and ability to think. It is also an antioxidant.

St John's Wort: This herb has been used for centuries to treat brain disorders and also promotes mental wellbeing. It is widely used in France and Germany in the treatment of depression.

Siberian Ginseng: This herb has a balancing effect on the neuro-transmitters in the brain. It is believed to help combat the symptoms of depression and stress, including mood swings, insomnia and tiredness.

Once you have been diagnosed and started treatment under the care of your doctor, it's time to turn to the pages of this book.

Starting to help yourself

If you are depressed, you probably feel your life is a shambles and you don't want to be bothered with anything. It may be an effort just to get up in the mornings, let alone carry on your everyday life. But rest assured, you can help yourself get through your depression by managing your life differently. The simplest way to achieve this is to make lists of short, easy tasks to do each day.

Take things slowly

Don't expect miracles and don't set yourself up to fail. Your illness could take some time to cure so it's important to set yourself goals you can reach. Take every day literally one step at a time. Have just small tasks to achieve each day. At the beginning, this may be just making sure you get fully dressed, brush your hair and clean your teeth.

Remember what you want to achieve

Remind yourself each morning what it is you want to achieve that day. Write post-it notes to yourself and stick them at strategic places to flag up anything that you want to try and do. Don't do many to start with and, again, keep it simple. This is the sort of thing I mean.

- Make the bed.
- Read the newspaper headlines.
- Read two articles of the newspaper.
- Call a friend or relative just to say hello.
- Sort out your underwear or sock drawer.
- Weed a small flowerbed or window box.
- File your nails.
- Write a letter or send an e-mail to a friend or relative.

One or two per day may be all you can manage to start with, then increase as you find you have more motivation. Don't try to do too many too soon, or you'll be disappointed and frustrated – which is not the idea.

As you achieve one, you can enjoy ceremoniously taking down its note. Don't throw them away. At the end of the day, you can see how many little goals you have achieved and over a period of time you should see this number rise.

Keep to small, manageable jobs

Don't give yourself large tasks. For instance, your home may be in an awful mess and need cleaning. Don't try and tackle the whole thing. Just do one bit at a time: vacuum the floor **or** dust the surfaces **or** hang up your clothes **or** clean the loo. Once that first task is completed you can do another one when you feel able, which may be that day or, perhaps, the next.

Eat properly

Easier said than done, I know, but there's plenty in this book to help you get all the right nutrients without having to make much effort at all. It is important, though; if you don't eat or eat poorly, you will definitely feel worse. So follow either the snack eating plan starting on page 39 or the three-meals-a-day plan on page 68.

Look after your appearance

Another hard one, especially when you probably think no one cares how you look. The point is, it will affect how you feel about yourself – and there's nothing more depressing than seeing your own bedraggled reflection in the mirror. So at the very least, try to put on some clean clothes each day and keep your hair clean and tidy.

Ask for help

Don't be afraid to ask friends or family for practical help – particularly with making sure you eat properly. Just someone checking what you are having for dinner could be enough to make you feel obliged to eat it!

If you can't face shopping, get a friend or relative to do it for you. Use the shopping list on page 133 as a guide or look at the eating plans in Chapters 8 and 9. They will help you to make the decisions about what needs to be bought.

Take some light exercise

Don't skip this one, no matter how sluggish you feel. Charlotte will explain all about it later in the book but suffice to say now that exercise will help to give you that 'feel-good' factor you need.

Don't hide yourself away

Try to get out and meet people. If you have family or friends, tell them about your illness. The old adage of 'a problem shared is a problem halved' really is true. Family and friends will want to help. If you are alone, you will feel lonely and unloved and all those negative thoughts will start to multiply. When you are with others, their positive attitude will begin to rub off.

Give yourself a break

If your depression is caused by the stress of your daily life, you may find that doing something creative will help you to unwind. It is interesting to note that people whose occupation involves long periods of intense intellectual activity involving dry facts and figures often find that an activity such as painting or sewing is a great help in relieving stress and depression. It doesn't matter how bad you are at it – as long as you enjoy the experience. So anxious accountants and medical students may discover that trying their hand at cookery, sketching or carpentry will help them to deal with their tension. It's certainly a better option than resorting to drink.

Postpone important decisions

Don't make any important decisions right now. Wait until you feel better.

Trust yourself – you will get better

Do believe you will soon feel a little better and that eventually the depression will disappear completely. It takes time, but gradually the black cloud will lift as your body responds to any medical help you are receiving and your self-help programme.

Be kind to yourself

This is very important. Many depressed people suffer from feelings of guilt, somehow blaming themselves for their illness and their apparent inability to 'snap out of it'. Try not to fall into this trap – it is not going to make things better and will certainly delay your recovery.

chapter four

How Food Can Help

I f you're like me, you won't feel like eating at all when you're depressed but you may find you 'comfort eat', usually junk food or chocolate, to try to ease the pain and misery. Either way, the unbalanced diet means you are actually depriving yourself of the very nutrients that can help you feel better.

Vitamins and minerals that will help

The list below gives details of the vitamins and minerals your body really needs to give you a sense of wellbeing and the foods that contain them.

- **B vitamins (especially folic acid and B6):** Found in vegetables, especially green leafy ones and potatoes, dried peas, beans and lentils, peanuts, eggs, fruit, nuts, whole grains, wholemeal bread, Marmite or other yeast extract, fish, offal (like liver and kidneys) and poultry.

- **Vitamin C:** Found in fruit and vegetables, particularly (bell) peppers, potatoes, citrus fruit, kiwi fruit, tomatoes, strawberries and blackcurrants.

- **Calcium:** Found in milk, cheese and other dairy products, green leafy vegetables, canned fish with bones, such as sardines (eat the bones too for a real boost!).

- **Potassium:** Found in avocados, dried peas, beans and lentils, nuts and seeds, dried fruit, tomatoes, fruit (particularly bananas and oranges) and wheatgerm.

- **Iron:** Found in offal, other meats, sardines, egg yolks, green leafy vegetables and fortified breakfast cereals.

- **Magnesium:** Found in dried peas, beans and lentils, nuts, seeds (particularly sesame seeds), dried figs, wheat germ and whole grains.

- **Copper:** Found in liver, shellfish, nuts, mushrooms and cocoa.

- **Zinc:** Found in shellfish (particularly oysters), whole grains, meat, poultry, eggs, dairy products, nuts, peanuts and seeds.

Later in the book you will find two easy-eating regimes that are both high in these nutrients, to help you feel better on a day-to-day basis. I have devised these to suit different eating habits. If you have been overeating and need to avoid comfort junk, or can't face big meals, I suggest you try the first eating plan, which starts on page 39. This is based on having a snack every couple of hours. If, however, you prefer to eat three meals a day, with just a tiny snack mid-afternoon, then the second plan, starting on page 68, is probably better suited to you. Both the plans use convenience foods to make life really easy for you, and I've topped these up with the nutrients you need to get your body back on track.

I have also included a range of easy-to make recipes at the back of the book to help you maintain your balanced diet when you're ready.

Foods to limit

As I have already said, there are some foods that will actually make your depression worse. These foods should only appear occasionally in your diet.

- Deep-fried and other fatty foods.

- Foods with a high sugar content: the odd piece of high-quality chocolate is good for you but don't eat loads of sweets (candies), sweet biscuits (cookies) or cakes.

- Caffeine: too much exacerbates the symptoms of depression so have no more than two cups a day and definitely none during the evening or before you go to bed. Choose caffeine-free tea, coffee and cola instead.

- Alcohol. You don't have to give it up altogether (unless you have a drink problem). If you enjoy an aperitif to stimulate your appetite or a glass of wine with your dinner, to make your meal more pleasurable, then continue to have one. Don't drink to excess, however, or you will make your symptoms much worse. Stick to no more than one or two small drinks a day. If you are on medication, check with your doctor if it is safe for you to drink.

Meals when on medication

Some medications cannot be taken with particular foods. If you have been prescribed monoamine oxidase inhibitors (MAOIs) for your depression, your doctor should give you a list of foods that you must avoid. These include many of the foods in my diet plans and, because of this, the plans could not be used without considerable modification.

If you are on MAOIs, the diet regime in this book is not suitable for you.

It is most important that you take any medication exactly as instructed by your doctor or pharmacist. Some medicines should be taken on an empty stomach; others should be taken with, or after, meals, so do read the directions carefully. Note also that some medications will 'clash' with each other. If you are on prescribed medication, always ask for advice before taking any over-the-counter remedies at the same time – including pills for common ailments, such as headaches and indigestion. If you aren't good at remembering to take your anti-depressants, pencil them in at the appropriate times in the diet and exercise regime you choose to use on page 39 or 68 as an added reminder.

If you are on any medication, always consult your doctor before embarking on a new dietary regime, including the ones in this book.

Planning healthy meals

It is very important that you eat regularly and well. If you don't, your blood-sugar levels will plummet and you will feel even more tired and listless. You don't have to have huge meals: you may find that having nutritious snacks is an easier way for you to get the nutrients you need without having to face full meals. If you have been binge-eating, the snack approach will help you too, because you are less likely to feel hungry in between.

Both of the meal plans I have devised will provide you with an easy, no-effort-required option – there's no need to think what you will eat, just read the plan you have chosen to follow, and go out and buy whatever you need for that day. Alternatively, you can look at the lists of suggested vital nutrients on page 24, decide on your own version of the snack plan or the full meals plan, and do it yourself. But either way, you must stick to your plan and follow it rigidly.

If cooking is on your list of 'can't face it' chores, you may find it best to prepare meals in advance, so that when it's time to eat, you only have to do the last-minute cooking (or just get the food out of the fridge). Always choose meals that involve the minimum of effort. If you know you will deliberately skip meals, try asking a friend or family member to help out. Show them the plan and they will gladly prepare something for you and encourage you to eat it.

If you choose to go for the three-meals-a-day plan starting on page 68, it means just that, so make sure you do have those **three meals** – breakfast, lunch and dinner – at the very least. You can have healthy extras in between, too, such as a piece of fresh fruit or a handful of pumpkin seeds or nuts and raisins.

If you can't face eating whole meals, follow the snack plan on page 39. But remember, you must have at least **six snacks** a day in place of meals.

Here are some helpful tips to make meal preparation less of an obstacle and to ensure that you always have food to hand.

- Make sure you have plenty of nutritious convenience foods in the house, from microwave rice to lasagne. Look at the shopping list in Chapter 12 and the tips for convenience food eating starting on page 28.

- Buy fresh fruit and vegetables regularly. Choose vegetables that need little preparation, like courgettes (zucchini), French (green) beans and broccoli. At extra expense – but worth it if you are really low – you can buy ready-prepared carrots, cabbage, salads and so on. Alternatively, buy frozen vegetables or cans (choose the varieties in natural juice or water).

- Keep sliced loaves of bread, rolls and a good range of other bread products in the freezer. Individual slices and everything from rolls to flour tortillas can be taken out as you need them, leaving the rest wrapped and frozen for other days. You can thaw them in just a few seconds under the grill (broiler) or in the microwave.

- Store a selection of easy-to-cook meats and fish in the freezer, such as chicken breasts, fish fillets and mince (ground meat). If buying fresh, go for steaks, chops and other individual items that can be cooked quickly with little preparation.

- Keep a good supply of nuts, seeds and dried fruit to hand for healthy nibbles.

If you have had a very low-fibre diet up till now – white bread and hardly any fresh fruit or vegetables – you may prefer to introduce this new regime gradually so it isn't so much of a shock to your system. So, for the first week, have white bread with added fibre instead of wholemeal, and substitute fresh fruit for the dried. The second week, you can have the dried fruit, and then in the third week, introduce the wholemeal bread too.

Make eating a pleasure

When preparing a meal, try to make it a pleasurable occasion: lay the table, preferably, or set up a tray. Arrange the knife and fork, give yourself a napkin – even if it's only a piece of kitchen paper (paper towel) – and fill an attractive drinking glass with water.

Make the meal look tempting – arrange it nicely, add a suitable garnish, like a sprig of parsley. Don't overdo the size of the portions. If you find a full plate of food daunting, try using a large plate, then arrange the portion of food attractively so it looks smaller. Alternatively, you could put a small portion on a small plate to avoid the danger of serving yourself too much.

Remember to drink plenty of water – six to eight glasses – throughout the day. It can be straight from the tap, bottled (still or sparkling), or even flavoured.

Tips on making ready meals healthy

It is highly unlikely that you are going to have the energy and inclination to spend ages cooking – which is where ready meals come in. However, they are not always very well balanced, and some are just plain dull. Worry not: here are some quick and simple tips to make them easier to prepare, tastier and more nutritious.

- If the dish should be served with rice, choose a brand that includes it with the other ingredients – such as Thai red curry with jasmine rice. If cooking your own, boil the rice rather than frying.

- Choose a dish that includes added vegetables.

- If you like Indian food, go for tandoori, plain tikkas or biryanis. Avoid curries in sauces – these tend to be packed with oil and cream, which you should avoid.

- Avoid parathas (deep-fried) and keema naans, which often contain processed meats.

- If you like Chinese, go for dishes that include noodles and lots of vegetables, such as chow mein.

- Do try to eat a separate vegetable (frozen or canned are easiest, but fresh is best if you can be bothered) with your ready meal. A bowl of salad is just as good and quick to prepare.

- Choose ready meals that can be steamed or microwaved. These are usually better for you than those that have to be baked in the oven.

- Pizza is the ultimate quick and easy meal. To ensure yours has the nutrients you need, choose a cheese and tomato one and add extra fresh toppings (see the meal plan on page 170) or buy one with lots of vegetables on it.

- Avoid meals laden with food colourings (especially bright red or yellow).

- Avoid deep-fried foods in batter – including the Chinese ones like sweet and sour pork, chicken or prawn balls.

- Avoid fried and oven-baked 'brown' snacks, such as spring rolls, samosas, etc.

chapter five

How Exercise Can Help

Y ou know that exercise is good for you physically, but you might not know that it may actually improve mental heath. There are a number of reasons for this.

- It gives you a feel-good factor. Regular exercise improves your physical appearance, enhances your mood and makes you look forward to your meals.

- Working your large muscle groups helps get rid of pent-up stress.

- It releases the chemicals in your brain (neurotransmitters) that regulate your mood. People suffering from depression have low levels of neurotransmitters, and so raising the levels will help improve their mood. One group, known as beta-endorphins, is known to reduce pain, regulate emotions and make you feel happier. When doing light to moderate exercise, the brain increases the amount of monoamines, too, which have an anti-depressant effect.

- Warming your body during exercise will naturally relieve stress.

- Exercise can act as a distraction or 'time out', which stops you thinking about your problems.

- Regular exercise builds your confidence as you find you are able to complete the specific tasks involved. This can carry over into other aspects of your life, and increase your sense of control, so helping relieve your symptoms even more.

- Exercise classes can add a social dimension to your life, helping you even more to overcome your depression.

What kind of exercise?

Exercise to combat depression does not need to be hard and exhausting; in fact it is very important that it is gentle and enjoyable. Ideally, any form of light to moderate aerobic exercise is a good idea. Walking is perfect. It doesn't need any special equipment, you can do it any time, anywhere, and it encourages you to get out into the fresh air. You only need to walk just a bit faster than normal – as though you are hurrying for the bus – for it to do you good. You could try jogging if you are feeling up to it, and swimming is another great way to exercise gently.

Other forms of exercise to tone you up, such as Pilates or working out with weights, can also make you feel great. You'll find everything you need to know in Chapter 10, All about Exercise. Alternatively, if you feel up to it, you could join a yoga, aerobics or dance class.

How often should I exercise?

You don't have to exercise every day. In fact, doing too much exercise may, actually, do more harm than good. Start off gently – twice a week – and build up gradually to three or perhaps four sessions. That doesn't mean you have to be a couch potato on those 'rest' days. Try to do some active tasks – such as a gentle stroll, or light housework or gardening – every day. These do not count towards your exercise regime, however.

How long should I exercise?

You should aim for 15–30 minutes at a time – just a short, brisk walk, perhaps, for a newspaper or to post a letter – but for no more than an hour at a time.

How long before I notice the effects?

Your exercise programme is an integral part of your whole self-help regime. Don't expect immediate results. The effects will be cumulative. You may get bursts of feeling great just because you are doing the programme but, in real terms, it will be between six and 10 weeks before you see real noticeable physiological and psychological changes.

chapter six

How to Get a Good Night's Sleep

....

When you are depressed – and possibly stressed as well – it is really important that you get enough rest and relaxation. That's easy to say, and you probably know it already, but it can be very hard to do when you lie awake at night knowing you are tired and need to sleep but are not able to switch off.

There are many things you can try to help you crack this problem. However, everyone responds differently, so you'll need to work your way through the options until you find something that helps you to switch off, relax and drift off comfortably. The most important thing is to create a relaxing routine for yourself to help you wind down before going to sleep.

- Have a warm, fragrant bath with soothing herbal oils or bubble bath. There are many commercial preparations available that have herbs already added. Alternatively, you can buy them individually or in combination as oils to put in your bath (see page 19 for more information).

- Try massaging relaxing aromatherapy oils into your temples and wrists. You can buy these ready-blended from your local chemist or health food shop. A small phial with a roller ball is great for rubbing on without mess.

- Listen to calming music. Choose something you enjoy – it can be anything from classical to folk ballads as long as it is soothing – or you could go for a special compilation CD.

- Dim the lights or use candles to soften the mood.

- Try eating a small bowl of oat porridge about an hour before bedtime. Oats are a natural anti-depressant and so may help to alleviate your night anxieties.

- Drink a warm milky drink or a herbal infusion, such as chamomile, valerian, passionflower, Californian poppy, peppermint or fennel.

- Make sure you have a comfortable pillow. An old lumpy one may give you a headache.

- Change your bedding frequently. Fresh, fragrant sheets are far more pleasant to get into than stale, grubby ones.

- Try putting a soft cushion or small pillow between your knees to increase your sense of comfort and wellbeing.

- Make sure you have the right amount of bedding. If you are too hot or too cold during the night, your sleep pattern will be impaired, so a number of layers that you can throw off or pull on is better than just a duvet.

- Make sure you have a drink of water by your bed to sip if you wake up.

- Go to the loo just before you retire to try to prevent having to get up in the night.

- Make sure your room is well ventilated but free from draughts.

- Have a pot plant near your bed – such as a Christmas cactus. It will help balance the air in your room and aid sleep.

- Make sure the light is right for you. If you like sleeping in the dark, make sure you have thick curtains. If you don't like darkness, have a nightlight on the landing or an illuminated plug that fits into the electric socket.

- Take a natural herbal sleep remedy at bedtime. These are available from all good pharmacies. Remember, **you must check with your doctor first if you are on medication**.

- Try a repetitive and relaxing ritual, such as counting sheep, to help you drop off.

If all else fails and you find you are exhausted during the day, you can always take a power nap after lunch – but not in the evening. This should be very short – 10 to 20 minutes is quite enough to refresh you without spoiling your ability to sleep at night. Set an alarm to make sure you don't sleep for longer.

There are other things to avoid.

- Don't eat a big meal in the evening. Have your main meal at lunchtime, or at least not later than 7 pm.

- Don't eat fatty foods at night.

- Don't be tempted to eat cheese or drink a caffeine-based drink (such as coffee or tea) during the evening.

- Don't drink alcohol before you go to bed – it acts as a stimulant not a sleep-inducer. Of course, if you drink a lot, it will make you pass out, but your natural sleep-pattern will be disturbed and you will probably wake up after a few hours, feeling worse than ever.

- Don't smoke – nicotine is also a stimulant.

- Don't listen to loud rock or dance music before bedtime.

- Don't watch a horror movie or a bloodthirsty thriller before you go to bed.

- Don't make emotional phone calls late at night.

- Don't allow yourself to fall asleep on the sofa before bedtime – there's no better way to take the edge off your sleepiness.

- Don't have a loud ticking clock by your bed. Choose a silent one. Avoid clocks with an illuminated face or you'll be tempted to keep checking the time if you can't sleep.

- Don't lie in late in the morning, even if you have had a bad night – this will only perpetuate the cycle, so get up on schedule and make a start to your day.

Tried-and-tested methods to get you back to sleep

Waking in the middle of the night is a classic symptom of depression. If this happens to you and you're unable to go back to sleep, try these methods to send you off again.

- Lie on your back, arms resting at your sides, eyes closed. Beginning with your head, start consciously relaxing your body. Feel each part becoming heavy, sinking into the softness of the mattress. Neck, shoulders, arms, back ... all the way down to your feet. All the time breathe slowly and regularly.

- Lie in your most comfortable sleeping position. With your eyes closed, 'look' deep into the darkness you see. Imagine the number one in your head. Concentrate on trying to see that number in your mind's eye. When – and only when – you can visualise the number one, pass on to the number two, then three ... Continue visualising numbers, one at a time. You probably won't get past 10, provided you don't cheat!

- Lie in your most comfortable sleeping position. Close your eyes and imagine you are pretending to be asleep. Deliberately slow your breathing right down. Don't move, just keep your eyes closed, feel relaxed and breathe very slowly and deeply.

- Lie in your most comfortable sleeping position. Close your eyes. Breathe slowly and deeply. Picture the sea, with the waves ebbing and flowing on the shore. The sea may be calm or rough – choose whichever pleases you most. The important thing is the rhythm of the waves. Try and actually see those waves in your mind's eye, watching each wave roll up the beach, then draw back into the sea as the next one breaks.

- Lie in your most comfortable sleeping position. Make a conscious effort not to think about anything in particular. Concentrate on the word 'sleep'. If you realise you are thinking anything at all, blank it out again and keep thinking 'sleep'. At the same time, breathe slowly, deeply and regularly.

- If all of the above fails, it is better to get up, make yourself a warm milky drink or herbal tea, and listen to some soothing music or read for a while. Then go back to bed and try again.

- Have a notepad and pen or pencil by your bed. If you wake and you find yourself worrying about all sorts of things – whether they are to do with your depression or not – you can write down what's bothering you. It's amazing how once it's all down on paper, you are able to put it out of your mind – even if only for the time being. In the same way, if you find yourself planning things you need to do or to act on the next day, write them down. This will free your mind ready to sleep – and avoids those clearly thought-out solutions in the middle of the night being muddled or forgotten in the morning!

chapter seven

Relaxing Tasks

I suggested in an earlier chapter that you do a small or relaxing task a couple of times a day. Relaxation is an almost-forgotten art for many people nowadays but it is vital to our health and wellbeing and this is all the more important if you are depressed.

The tasks that you choose should not only relax you but also give you a sense of achievement; this is important in how you feel you have done during that day. No one can tell you what you find relaxing – the idea of doing a quick crossword, for example, is one person's idea of fun and another's idea of mental torture – so take a look at the list of suggestions on the next couple of pages, cross out those you would not enjoy and add your own favourites.

When you have a little 'down' time, go through your personalised list, and choose a task that you like the look of. Don't do the same thing every time – work your way through the list so you get variety in your activities. And remember, the aim here is relaxation, so don't go for anything that is too taxing.

- **Read a book:** Don't pick anything too long or involved; this is probably not the moment to tackle *War and Peace*!
  Re-reading a favourite book, or one you have read before, is a good idea as it doesn't demand so much from your memory and concentration. Alternatively, you could read a children's book. Many adult books are just too much like hard work when your concentration is shot, so a children's book will be entertaining but less demanding. I would recommend the Harry Potter series, for example, or something by Jacqueline Wilson or Terry Pratchett.

- **Flick through a magazine:** Because the information is presented in small pieces, magazines are less taxing than books. Concentrate only on the pictures if that's all you can manage, or decide to read only one article.

- **Read a newspaper or a supplement:** Even if you usually read the *Financial Times*, opt for something a bit easier to absorb.

- **Read a periodical:** If it worries you that you are getting out of touch with work, you may find it helpful to read an article in a professional journal.

- **Do a crossword:** Again, even if you are usually a *Daily Telegraph* expert, don't expect to perform at your best. You may have to change to something simpler for a while.

- **Try a word or number puzzle:** Word searches, sudoku and other puzzles can be fun but do choose easy ones.

- **Do some knitting, crochet, cross stitch, patchwork or sewing:** Choose a simple project, not a major one.

- **Do some gardening:** Don't try to revamp your herbaceous border – just clear some leaves or do a bit of weeding or tidying.

- **Draw or paint:** You don't have to be good – you don't even have to show anyone – but it can be relaxing.

- **Listen to music:** Your choice of music can seriously affect your mood so choose wisely: something either invigorating or calming but not depressing.

- **Watch TV:** Check the listings and find something you really enjoy.

- **Watch a video or DVD:** If your concentration is poor, don't try to watch a full-length film, opt for something you have taped, such as a game of sport, or an episode of one of your favourite comedy or drama shows.

- **Listen to the radio:** Look out for comedy programmes, travel, or something on a topic that interests you.

- **Look through a recipe book:** If you feel a growing interest in food, browse through one of your favourite recipe books and choose a recipe or two you'd like to try out.

- **Bake a cake:** It doesn't take a lot of effort to make a few muffins or a simple cake, the smell will be delicious and you can give yourself a treat.

- **Groom the dog or cat:** Stroking motions are very therapeutic and as long as your pet enjoys the experience, you will both benefit.

- **Wash and style your hair:** Concentrating on making yourself look your best can enhance your mood.

- **Manicure your nails:** Soak your hands in warm water, then take your time to smooth on plenty of hand cream and file your nails, then paint them if you like.

- **Give yourself a pedicure:** Try a hot soak, scrub, soften with hand or foot cream and trim your toenails.

- **Do a jigsaw.**

- **Have a game of patience.**

- **Go for a walk:** Just a gentle amble, purely for the enjoyment.

- **Take a few photographs:** Go to the park, or just take some snaps in your garden or your street.

It is quite likely that, having made a list, you find it hard to choose something to do. If so, choose the first thing on the list that you know you would have enjoyed before your illness and define exactly what you are going to do: one row of knitting, four newspaper headlines, walk to the post box on the corner. That will help you to progress.

If you really feel you could not care less about doing anything at all, it is advisable to go back to your doctor, or to visit him or her if you have not already done so. You do need to be properly diagnosed and they can help you to get past this block.

chapter eight

Your Two-week, Six-snacks-a-day Diet and Exercise Plan

his snack plan is designed for those of you who hate big meals. The idea is that you eat little and often, giving your body all the nutrients you need in small portions. In the same way, I have divided each day into short periods, with exercise sessions and household tasks incorporated into the daily plan. This assumes, of course, that your depression is severe enough to prevent you from working at the moment. But if you are still trying to carry on working as normal, then it will probably be easier for you to follow the three-meals-a-day plan on page 68, fitting it in with your daily commitments.

When you have completed two weeks on this plan, if you feel you are ready, move on to the rest of the exercise programme table in Chapter 10. Continue to follow this same diet plan or, if you prefer, go on to the three-meals a day one on page 68 and repeat these two-week cycles for the next eight weeks. If you choose to stay on the snack plan, don't allow yourself to slip into bad habits – keep avoiding those sugary, fatty junk foods.

After eight weeks on the programme, you will probably find that you are feeling much better. To maintain this improvement, I would suggest that you continue with the exercise programme and, instead of the diet plans, try the range of delicious, nutritious maintenance recipes at the back of the book.

Super-fast snack

If you have a microwave and really can't summon the enthusiasm for anything fancy, here is my top tip for a nutritious lunch or supper.

Beany stuffed jacket-baked potato

Prick a large scrubbed potato all over with a fork. Wrap in a piece of kitchen paper (paper towel) and microwave on High for 4–5 minutes until really soft. Split open the potato, then spoon on a small can of baked beans in tomato sauce and add a handful of grated Cheddar cheese. Microwave for a further 1–2 minutes until hot and the cheese has melted.

Tips on using the programme

Drink plenty of water during the day. You can also enjoy cups of decaffeinated tea or coffee, sugar-free soft drinks or glasses of skimmed or semi-skimmed milk as you feel like it. Avoid fizzy drinks as they will fill you up.

If you feel hungry at any time, you can always add in an extra snack (ideally fresh or dried fruit, nuts and seeds or low-fat carbohydrates, like a plain currant bun or teacake, or a bread roll or crispbread with your favourite low-fat/low-sugar filling or topping).

You don't have to actually make up the snack meal suggestions – just eat all the ingredients. So, for example, if you can't even be bothered to make the Beef and Horseradish Wrap on page 62, simply fold the tortilla, and eat it with the slices of cold beef, a tomato, a chunk of cucumber and a wedge of lettuce.

You can swap any snack meal with a similar one from another day – or even whole days, if you like – and you can also substitute any fruit for another one. Also, if you like only one of the days' suggestions, eat those snack meals every day – but beware of boredom, as it won't help to lift your mood.

I've suggested specific times for everything you do, but these are only intended as a guideline. They can be as flexible as you want them to be. I know, for instance, it doesn't take an hour to eat a banana! The idea is that, during that time, you will eat the banana, maybe listening to the radio or whatever, and continue doing the other activities suggested when you have finished. The important thing is to eat little and often, incorporating your exercises and tasks in the day.

Day 1

7–8 am	Get up, make a cup of decaffeinated tea or coffee, have a wash and get dressed (you can dress after breakfast if you prefer).
8–9 am	Prepare and eat breakfast. **A glass of pure fruit juice** **A bowl of wholegrain cereal with milk and a handful of raisins**
9–10 am	Clear up breakfast. Have a shower and dress, if you have not already done so. Set yourself a task to do now – like making your bed. Set some tasks for later and write them on post-it notes to stick around as reminders.
10–11 am	Have a snack. **A banana**
11 am–12 noon	Aerobic exercise. Walk, jog, cycle or swim for 15 minutes (see Chapter 10). Freshen up.
12 noon–1 pm	Prepare and eat lunch. **$1/2$ large or 1 small avocado, stoned (pitted) with a spoonful of cottage cheese, a handful of chopped walnuts, a squeeze of lemon juice and a good grinding of black pepper** **1 rye or other wholegrain crispbread (optional)**
1–2 pm	Clear up lunch. Have a power nap for 20 minutes, if you feel tired. If not, read the newspaper or a book, or sit quietly and listen to some music.
2–3 pm	Have a snack. **An oatcake with a finger of cheese** **A tomato**
3–4 pm	Do another small task or visit or entertain a friend.
4–5 pm	Have a snack. **A fruit yoghurt** **Some pieces of fresh fruit**
5–6 pm	Read a magazine, or a book if you are up to it, or other relaxing task.

6–7 pm   Prepare and eat your supper.
              Ham and salad sandwich (see recipe box)

Ham and salad sandwich
Spread two slices of wholemeal bread with a little butter or low-fat spread. Fill with slices of ham, a sliced tomato, some sliced cucumber, a couple of lettuce leaves, a spoonful of mayonnaise and a little mustard.

---

7 pm–bedtime Check how many 'achieving' tasks you've managed by looking at your post-it notes. Relax by watching TV or a DVD, read a book, do a crossword, etc. Follow the suggestions on 'How to Get a Good Night's Sleep' (see page 32).

Day 2

7–8 am	Get up, make a cup of decaffeinated tea or coffee, have a wash and get dressed (you can dress after breakfast if you prefer).
8–9 am	Prepare and eat breakfast. **A glass of pure fruit juice** **A bowl of instant hot oat porridge made with milk and a teaspoon of clear honey**
9–10 am	Clear up breakfast. Have a shower and dress, if not already done. Choose a task to do now. Set some tasks for later and write them on post-it notes.
10–11 am	Have a snack. **A handful of dried apricots**
11 am–12 noon	Light exercise. Go for a gentle, not brisk, walk or do some other light exercise, like some gardening. Freshen up.
12 noon–1 pm	Prepare and eat lunch. **Baked beans on wholemeal toast, topped with a handful of grated Cheddar cheese**
1–2 pm	Clear up lunch. Have a power nap for 20 minutes, if tired. If not, read the newspaper or a book.
2–3 pm	Have a snack. **An apple and two squares (no more) of good-quality chocolate with 70 per cent cocoa solids**
3–4 pm	Do another small task or visit or entertain a friend.
4–5 pm	Have a snack. **A toasted crumpet with a little peanut butter and/or a teaspoon of raspberry jam (conserve)**
5–6 pm	Read a book or magazine.

6–7 pm   Prepare and eat your supper.
Tuna and sweetcorn salad (see recipe box)
A wholegrain roll (optional)

Tuna and sweetcorn salad
Mix some salad leaves from a ready-prepared pack with some sliced tomato, cucumber and red or green (bell) pepper. Top with a small can of tuna, drained, half a small can of sweetcorn and a dollop of mayonnaise or a sprinkling of French dressing.

Note: Put the rest of the corn in a covered container in the fridge for Day 4.

---

7 pm–bedtime   Relax: watch TV or a DVD, read a book, do a crossword, etc. Follow the suggestions on 'How to Get a Good Night's Sleep' (see page 32).

Day 3

7–8 am	Get up, make a cup of decaffeinated tea or coffee, have a wash and get dressed (you may dress after breakfast if you prefer).
8–9 am	Prepare and eat breakfast. **A glass of pure fruit juice** **A bowl of muesli with milk**
9–10 am	Clear up breakfast. Have a shower and dress, if not already done. Choose a task to do now. Set some tasks for later and write them on post-it notes to stick around as reminders.
10–11 am	Have a snack. **A banana**
11 am–12 noon	Light exercise. Go for a gentle, not brisk, walk or do some light housework, like vacuuming, if you feel like it. Do another task, if you have time.
12 noon–1 pm	Prepare and eat lunch. **Wholemeal pitta breads cut into fingers, with hummus** **1 small courgette (zucchini) and ¹/₂ red (bell) pepper, cut into strips**
1–2 pm	Clear up lunch. Have a power nap for 20 minutes, if tired. If not, read the newspaper or a book.
2–3 pm	Have a snack. **An apple with a small piece of cheese**
3–4 pm	Do another small task or visit or entertain a friend.
4–5 pm	Have a snack. **A fruit and nut cereal bar**
5–6 pm	Choose a relaxing task, such as reading.
6–7 pm	Prepare and eat your supper. **A can of chicken and vegetable soup (or other similar soup of your choice with lots of vegetables), with some canned sweetcorn added** **A granary bread roll with butter or low-fat spread**
7 pm–bedtime	Relax: watch TV or a DVD, read a book, do a crossword, etc. Follow the suggestions on 'How to Get a Good Night's Sleep' (see page 32).

Day 4

7–8 am	Get up, make a cup of decaffeinated tea or coffee, have a wash and get dressed (dress after breakfast if you prefer).
8–9 am	Prepare and eat breakfast. **A glass of pure fruit juice** **A bowl of wholegrain breakfast cereal, with milk and a handful of pumpkin seeds and dried blueberries**
9–10 am	Clear up breakfast. Have a shower and dress, if not already done. Choose a task to do now. Set some tasks for later and write them on post-it notes to stick around as reminders.
10–11 am	Have a snack. **A pear**
11 am–12 noon	Exercise. Do a 20-minute toning or resistance/weight training routine, for upper body if using weights (see page 107 or 117). Freshen up.
12 noon– 1 pm	Prepare and eat lunch. **2 fish fingers, grilled (broiled), in a soft bread roll, with mayonnaise and lots of lettuce**
1–2 pm	Clear up lunch. Have a power nap for 20 minutes, if tired. If not, read the newspaper or a book.
2–3 pm	Have a snack. **A hazelnut (filbert) yoghurt**
3–4 pm	Do another small task or visit or invite a friend round.
4–5 pm	Have a snack. **A plain currant bun or teacake**
5–6 pm	Read a book or other relaxing task.

6–7 pm   Prepare and eat supper.
                 One or two cooked chicken legs with some watercress or mixed salad leaves
                 A walnut and orange salad (see recipe box)
                 Wholegrain crackers (optional)

Walnut and orange salad
Peel and segment a satsuma or clementine and put in a bowl. Chop a celery stick and add with a handful of walnuts. Mix with a tablespoon of mayonnaise.

---

7 pm–bedtime   Relax: watch TV or a DVD, read a book, do a crossword, etc. Follow the suggestions on 'How to Get a Good Night's Sleep' (see page 32).

Day 5

7–8 am	Get up, make a cup of decaffeinated tea or coffee, have a wash and get dressed (dress after breakfast if you prefer).
8–9 am	Prepare and eat breakfast. **A glass of pure fruit juice** **A bowl of wholegrain cereal with milk and a handful of grapes**
9–10 am	Clear up breakfast. Have a shower and dress, if not already done. Choose a task to do now. Set some tasks for later and write them on post-it notes to stick around as reminders.
10–11 am	Have a snack. **Half a small orange-fleshed melon, with a sprinkling of ground ginger (optional)**
11 am–12 noon	Light exercise. Go for a gentle, not brisk, walk or do some other gentle exercise, like some gardening. Freshen up.
12 noon–1 pm	Prepare and eat lunch. **Tomatoes and ham on toast** (see recipe box)

Tomatoes and ham on toast
Toast a slice of wholemeal bread under the grill (broiler) and add a little butter or low-fat spread. Top the toast with sliced ham, then sliced tomatoes and grill (broil) for 1–2 minutes to heat through. Sprinkle with a few drops of Worcestershire sauce, if liked, before serving.

1–2 pm	Have a power nap for 20 minutes, if tired. If not, read the newspaper or a book.
2–3 pm	Have a snack. **A fruit yoghurt** **Some pieces of fresh fruit**
3–4 pm	Do another small task, or see a friend.

4–5 pm	Have a snack. **A digestive biscuit (graham cracker) with a little peanut butter**
5–6 pm	Read a book or other relaxing task.
6–7 pm	Prepare and eat your supper. **A can of lentil or minestrone soup with a handful of grated cheese sprinkled on top** **A granary bread roll**
7 pm–bedtime	Relax: watch TV or a DVD, read a book, do a crossword, etc. Follow the suggestions on 'How to Get a Good Night's Sleep' (see page 32).

Day 6

7–8 am	Get up, make a cup of decaffeinated tea or coffee, have a wash and get dressed (dress after breakfast if you prefer).
8–9 am	Prepare and eat your breakfast. **A glass of pure fruit juice** **A bowl of hot instant oat cereal made with milk and a handful of raisins**
9–10 am	Clear up breakfast. Have a shower and dress, if not already done. Choose a task to do now. Set some tasks for later and write them on post-it notes to stick around as reminders.
10–11 am	Have a snack. **A banana**
11 am–12 noon	Light exercise. Go for a gentle, not brisk, walk, or do some other light exercise, such as gardening. Freshen up and do another task, if you have time.
12 noon–1 pm	Prepare and eat your lunch. **Chicken and cranberry wrap** (see recipe box) **Celery sticks (optional)**

Chicken and cranberry wrap

Heat a small can of chicken in white sauce in a saucepan (or use half a large can and store the rest in a covered container in the fridge and have it again tomorrow).

Spread a flour tortilla with a spoonful of cranberry sauce, then add some rocket, baby spinach, watercress or mixed salad leaves. Spread the hot chicken over, then roll up.

1–2 pm	Clear up lunch. Have a power nap for 20 minutes, if tired. If not, read the newspaper or a book.
2–3 pm	Have a snack. **An apple and two squares (no more) of good-quality chocolate with 70 per cent cocoa solids**
3–4 pm	Do another small task or visit or entertain a friend.

4–5 pm	Have a snack.
	A slice of wholemeal toast with a little butter or low-fat spread and Marmite or other yeast extract
5–6 pm	Relax by reading a book or other relaxing task.
6–7 pm	Prepare and eat your supper.
	Rosti with egg and tomato (see recipe box)

Rosti with egg and tomato

Heat the grill (broiler). Put a frozen potato rosti on a piece of foil on the rack and grill (broil) for 5 minutes.

Meanwhile, smear a little butter or low-fat spread in a ramekin dish (custard cup). Break an egg into the dish.

Halve a tomato. Turn the rosti over and put the egg and the halved tomato beside it. Grill for a further 3 minutes or until the rosti is golden, the egg is set and the tomato cooked. Cook a little longer if you like your egg hard.

Transfer the rosti and tomato to a plate. Either loosen the edge of the egg and turn it out on to the plate or eat it straight from the dish.

---

7 pm–bedtime	Relax: watch TV or a DVD, read a book, do a crossword, etc. Follow the wind-down suggestions on 'How to Get a Good Night's Sleep' (see page 32).

Day 7

7–8 am	Get up, make a cup of decaffeinated tea or coffee, have a wash and get dressed (dress after breakfast if you prefer).
8–9 am	Prepare and eat your breakfast. **A glass of pure fruit juice** **A small can of apricots in natural juice, topped with a small carton of apricot yoghurt and a crushed Weetabix**
9–10 am	Clear up breakfast. Have a shower and dress, if not already done. Choose a task to do now. Set some tasks for later and write them on post-it notes to stick around as reminders.
10–11 am	Have a snack. **A rye or wholegrain crispbread topped with a little peanut butter and sliced cucumber**
11 am–12 noon	Light exercise. Go for a gentle, not brisk, walk or do some similar exercise. Freshen up and do another task.
12 noon–1 pm	Prepare and eat your lunch. **Canned sardines on wholemeal toast** **Sliced tomato**
1–2 pm	Clear up lunch. Have a power nap for 20 minutes, if tired. If not, read the newspaper or a book.
2–3 pm	Have a snack. **An apple and two squares (no more) of good-quality chocolate with 70 per cent cocoa solids**
3–4 pm	Do another small task or visit or entertain a friend.
4–5 pm	Have a snack. **A toasted crumpet or teacake with a little butter or low-fat spread**
5–6 pm	Read a book or do some other relaxing task.

6–7 pm   Prepare and eat your supper.
Italian platter (see recipe box)
Ciabatta or other bread (optional)

Italian platter

Arrange slices of Parma or other raw cured ham, a quartered tomato, a handful of black or green olives, a handful of rocket, some Mozzarella, cut into bite-sized pieces, and a piece of orange-fleshed melon on a plate.

Trickle a little olive oil over and add a few drops of balsamic vinegar and a few torn fresh basil leaves, if you like.

---

7 pm–bedtime   Relax: watch TV or a DVD, read a book, do a crossword, etc. Follow the wind-down suggestions on 'How to Get a Good Night's Sleep' (see page 32).

Day 8

7–8 am	Get up, make a cup of decaffeinated tea or coffee, have a wash and get dressed (dress after breakfast if you prefer).
8–9 am	Prepare and eat your breakfast. **A glass of pure fruit juice** **A Weetabix, spread with butter or low-fat spread and marmalade**
9–10 am	Clear up breakfast. Have a shower and dress, if not already done. Choose a task to do now. Set some tasks for later and write them on post-it notes to stick around as reminders.
10–11 am	Have a snack. **A pear**
11 am–12 noon	Aerobic exercise. Walk, jog, cycle or swim for 15 minutes (see Chapter 10). Freshen up.
12 noon–1 pm	Prepare and eat your lunch. **Curried bean couscous** (see recipe box) **Celery sticks or chunks of cucumber**

Curried bean couscous

Put half a small mugful of couscous in a saucepan and add a small mugful of boiling water. Stir and leave to stand for 5 minutes until the liquid is absorbed.

Stir in a small can of baked beans in tomato sauce, a teaspoon of curry paste, a small handful of raisins and some salt and pepper. Cook over a gentle heat for about 2 minutes until really thick.

Tip into a bowl, add a few cubes of Cheddar cheese. Mix gently and serve before the cheese melts completely.

1–2 pm	Clear up lunch. Have a power nap for 20 minutes, if tired. If not, read the newspaper or a book.
2–3 pm	Have a snack. **An orange or two satsumas or clementines**

3–4 pm	Do another small task or visit or entertain a friend.
4–5 pm	Have a snack. **A slice of wholemeal toast with a little butter or low-fat spread and Marmite or other yeast extract**
5–6 pm	Read a book or other relaxing task.
6–7 pm	Prepare and eat your supper. **A slice of ready-made quiche** **A mixed salad with a little French dressing**
7 pm–bedtime	Relax: watch TV or a DVD, read a book, do a crossword, etc. Follow the wind-down suggestions on 'How to Get a Good Night's Sleep' (see page 32).

Day 9

7–8 am	Get up, make a cup of decaffeinated tea or coffee, have a wash and get dressed (dress after breakfast if you prefer).
8–9 am	Prepare and eat your breakfast. **A glass of pure fruit juice** **Mushrooms on toast** (see recipe box)

Mushrooms on toast

Heat a small can of mushrooms. Toast a slice of wholemeal bread and add a little butter or low-fat spread. Drain the mushrooms and put on top.

Sprinkle with dried oregano before serving.

9–10 am	Clear up breakfast. Have a shower and dress, if not already done. Choose a task to do now. Set some tasks for later and write them on post-it notes to stick around as reminders.
10–11 am	Have a snack. **A small carton of plain yoghurt with a teaspoonful of clear honey and a handful of sunflower seeds**
11 am–12 noon	Light exercise. Go for a gentle, not brisk, walk. Freshen up and do another task.
12 noon–1 pm	Prepare and eat your lunch. **Banana and date snackwich** (see recipe box)

Banana and date snackwich

Butter two slices of wholemeal bread. Mash a small banana. Spread on one buttered slice and top with a small handful of chopped dates and a small handful of desiccated (shredded) coconut. Cover with other slice of bread. Press down and cut into halves.

1–2 pm	Clear up lunch. Have a power nap for 20 minutes, if tired. If not, read the newspaper or a book.
2–3 pm	Have a snack. **An apple and two squares (no more) of good-quality chocolate with 70 per cent cocoa solids**
3–4 pm	Do another small task or visit or entertain a friend.
4–5 pm	Have a snack. **A wholegrain crispbread with a little butter or low-fat spread and Marmite or other yeast extract**
5–6 pm	Read a book or other relaxing task.
6–7 pm	Prepare and eat your supper. **Peanut soup** (see recipe box) **Cheese on wholemeal toast, with a few drops of Worcestershire sauce (optional)**

Peanut soup

Put a tablespoon of peanut butter in a mug. Add a sachet of instant chicken and vegetable soup. Fill the mug with boiling water, stirring all the time.

---

7 pm–bedtime	Relax: watch TV or a DVD, read a book, do a crossword, etc. Follow the suggestions on 'How to Get a Good Night's Sleep' (see page 32).

Day 10

7–8 am	Get up, make a cup of decaffeinated tea or coffee, have a wash and get dressed (dress after breakfast if you prefer).
8–9 am	Prepare and eat your breakfast. **A glass of pure fruit juice** **A small can of prunes or breakfast compôte in natural juice, warmed or cold, topped with a carton of plain yoghurt and a tablespoon of wheatgerm**
9–10 am	Clear up breakfast. Have a shower and dress, if not already done. Choose a task to do now. Set some tasks for later and write them on post-it notes to stick around as reminders.
10–11 am	Have a snack. **An oatcake and a small piece of cheese**
11 am–12 noon	Aerobic exercise. Walk, jog, cycle or swim for 15 minutes (see Chapter 10). Freshen up.
12 noon–1 pm	Prepare and eat your lunch. **Spicy dip with naan** (see recipe box) **Sticks of cucumber**

Spicy dip with naan

Heat a small can of pease pudding in a saucepan with two teaspoons of curry powder or paste, and a tablespoon of mango chutney or sweet pickle.

Warm a naan bread in the toaster, microwave or under the grill (broiler). Spoon the pea mixture on to the naan.

1–2 pm	Clear up lunch. Have a power nap for 20 minutes, if tired. If not, read the newspaper or a book.
2–3 pm	Have a snack. **A kiwi fruit**
3–4 pm	Do another small task or visit or entertain a friend.

4–5 pm	Have a snack. **A handful of peanuts or mixed nuts and raisins**
5–6 pm	Read a book or other relaxing task.
6–7 pm	Prepare and eat your supper. **Macaroni cheese with spinach** (see recipe box) **A sliced tomato**

Macaroni cheese with spinach
Heat a handful of chopped frozen spinach in a saucepan until thawed. Drain off any liquid. Stir in a small can of macaroni cheese and heat through.

---

7 pm–bedtime	Relax: watch TV or a DVD, read a book, do a crossword, etc. Follow the suggestions on 'How to Get a Good Night's Sleep' (see page 32).

Day 11

7–8 am	Get up, make a cup of decaffeinated tea or coffee, have a wash and get dressed (dress after breakfast if you prefer).
8–9 am	Prepare and eat your breakfast. **A glass of pure fruit juice** **A bowl of hot instant oat cereal, made with milk, mixed with a handful of dried blueberries**
9–10 am	Clear up breakfast. Have a shower and dress, if not already done. Choose a task to do now – like clearing up your room. Set some tasks for later and write them on post-it notes to stick around as reminders.
10–11 am	Have a snack. **An apple**
11 am–12 noon	Light exercise. Go for a gentle, not brisk, walk. Freshen up and do another task.
12 noon–1 pm	Prepare and eat your lunch. **BLT** (see recipe box)

BLT

Grill (broil) two slices of back bacon. Spread two slices of wholemeal bread with a little butter or low-fat spread.

Sandwich the bread together with the bacon, a sliced tomato, lots of crisp lettuce and a good spoonful of mayonnaise. Add a good grinding of black pepper too.

1–2 pm	Clear up lunch. Have a power nap for 20 minutes, if tired. If not, read the newspaper or a book.
2–3 pm	Have a snack. **A wedge of orange-fleshed melon with a pinch of ground ginger (optional)**
3–4 pm	Do another small task or visit or entertain a friend.

4–5 pm	Have a snack. **A handful of peanuts or mixed nuts and raisins**
5–6 pm	Read a book or other relaxing task.
6–7 pm	Prepare and eat your supper. **Italian cheese and tomato soup** (see recipe box) **A wholegrain bread roll or some crusty bread**

Italian cheese and tomato soup
Empty a small can of cream of tomato soup into a saucepan. Add a small can of chopped tomatoes. Heat through thoroughly, stirring. Add a handful of grated Mozzarella cheese and a good pinch of dried basil.

---

7 pm–bedtime	Relax: watch TV or a DVD, read a book, do a crossword, etc. Follow the suggestions on 'How to Get a Good Night's Sleep' (see page 32).

Day 12

7–8 am	Get up, make a cup of decaffeinated tea or coffee, have a wash and get dressed (dress after breakfast if you prefer).
8–9 am	Prepare and eat your breakfast. **A glass of pure fruit juice** **A banana and a glass of milk**
9–10 am	Clear up breakfast. Have a shower and dress, if not already done. Choose a task to do now – like clearing up your room. Set some tasks for later and write them on post-it notes to stick around as reminders.
10–11 am	Have a snack. **A slice of wholemeal toast with a little Marmite or other yeast extract**
11 am–12 noon	Exercise. Do a 20-minute resistance/weight training routine, for lower body if using weights (see page 107 or 117). Freshen up and do another task.
12 noon–1 pm	Prepare and eat your lunch. **Roast beef and horseradish wrap** (see recipe box)

Roast beef and horseradish wrap
Spread a flour tortilla with a little horseradish sauce, then a good spoonful of mayonnaise. Top with two slices of cold roast beef, some shredded lettuce and a grated carrot or a chopped tomato. Roll up.

1–2 pm	Clear up lunch. Have a power nap for 20 minutes, if tired. If not, read the newspaper or a book.
2–3 pm	Have a snack. **An apple and two squares (no more) of good-quality chocolate with 70 per cent cocoa solids**
3–4 pm	Do another small task or visit or entertain a friend.

4–5 pm	Have a snack. **Two dried apricots and a handful of pumpkin or sunflower seeds**
5–6 pm	Read a book or other relaxing task.
6–7 pm	Prepare and eat your supper. **Vegetable ravioli with peas** (see recipe box)

Vegetable ravioli with peas

Cook a good handful of frozen peas in a little water for 3–4 minutes until just tender. Drain and return to the pan. Add a can of vegetable ravioli and heat through. Tip into a bowl and top with a good handful of grated cheese (you can do this in the microwave if you like).

---

7 pm–bedtime	Relax: watch TV or a DVD, read a book, do a crossword, etc. Follow the suggestions on 'How to Get a Good Night's Sleep' (see page 32).

Day 13

7–8 am	Get up, make a cup of decaffeinated tea or coffee, have a wash and get dressed (dress after breakfast if you prefer).
8–9 am	Prepare and eat your breakfast. **A glass of pure fruit juice** **A bowl of wholegrain cereal with milk, a handful of sunflower seeds and raisins**
9–10 am	Clear up breakfast. Have a shower and dress, if not already done. Set yourself a task to do now – like clearing up your room. Set some tasks for later and write them on post-it notes to stick around as reminders.
10–11 am	Have a snack. **A kiwi fruit**
11 am–12 noon	Light exercise. Go for a gentle, not brisk, walk. Freshen up and do another task.
12 noon–1 pm	Prepare and eat your lunch. **One or two boiled eggs** **Wholemeal toast with a little butter or low-fat spread and Marmite or other yeast extract**
1–2 pm	Clear up lunch. Have a power nap for 20 minutes, if tired. If not, read the newspaper or a book.
2–3 pm	Have a snack. **Two plums**
3–4 pm	Do another small task or visit or entertain a friend.
4–5 pm	Have a snack. **A digestive biscuit (graham cracker) with a small piece of cheese** **A tomato or small bunch of grapes**
5–6 pm	Read a book or other relaxing task.

6–7 pm   Prepare and eat your supper.
                  Instant chilli bean soup (see recipe box)
                  A flour tortilla (optional)

Instant chilli bean soup
Empty a small can of cream of tomato soup into a saucepan. Add a pinch of chilli powder and a small can of baked beans in tomato sauce. Cook, stirring, until piping hot. Top with a handful of grated cheese.

---

7 pm–bedtime   Relax: watch TV or a DVD, read a book, do a crossword, etc. Follow the suggestions on 'How to Get a Good Night's Sleep' (see page 32).

Day 14

7–8 am	Get up, make a cup of decaffeinated tea or coffee, have a wash and get dressed (dress after breakfast if you prefer).
8–9 am	Prepare and eat your breakfast. **A glass of pure fruit juice** **A bowl of muesli with milk**
9–10 am	Clear up breakfast. Have a shower and dress, if not already done. Choose a task to do now. Set some tasks for later and write them on post-it notes to stick around as reminders.
10–11 am	Have a snack. **A slice of wholemeal toast with a little butter or low-fat spread and peanut butter**
11 am–12 noon	Light exercise. Go for a gentle, not brisk, walk. Freshen up and do another task.
12 noon–1 pm	Prepare and eat your lunch. **Egg mayonnaise** (see recipe box) **A wholegrain bread roll**

Egg mayonnaise
Boil one or two eggs in water for 5 minutes. Drain and cover with cold water.
   Shell the eggs and put on a bed of mixed salad leaves with some halved cherry tomatoes. Spoon some mayonnaise over.

1–2 pm	Clear up lunch. Have a power nap for 20 minutes, if tired. If not, read the newspaper or a book.
2–3 pm	Have a snack. **An orange or two satsumas or clementines**
3–4 pm	Do another small task or visit or entertain a friend.
4–5 pm	Have a snack. **A plain yoghurt with a handful of sunflower seeds and a teaspoon of clear honey**

5–6 pm   Read a book or other relaxing task.

6–7 pm   Prepare and eat your supper.
Minced beef topper (see recipe box)
A sliced tomato

Minced beef topper
Heat a small can of minced (ground) beef and onions with a tablespoon of tomato ketchup (catsup), a handful of frozen peas and a good pinch of dried oregano. Allow to bubble for 3 minutes, stirring frequently.

Toast a slice of wholemeal bread, add a little butter or low-fat spread, put on a plate and spoon the beef mixture on top.

---

7 pm–bedtime   Relax: watch TV or a DVD, read a book, do a crossword, etc. Follow the suggestions on 'How to Get a Good Night's Sleep' (see page 32).

chapter nine

Your Two-week,
Three-meals-a-day
Diet and Exercise Plan

· ·

T his chapter contains a complete guide to get you through the whole day from the moment you get up until you go to sleep at night. Although I have suggested entire menus, based on three meals per day, this does not involve lots of cooking because it uses ready meals with some simple extra ingredients to make them more healthy and appetising.

As in the snack plan in the previous chapter, this plan also includes a programme of simple exercises to fit into your day. When you have completed this two week plan, then continue with the same eating plan but go to the exercise plan in the table on page 131, which you can follow for the next eight weeks, incorporating it into this eating regime on the appropriate days.

Tips on following the programme

Drink plenty of water during the day. You can also enjoy cups of decaffeinated tea or coffee, sugar-free soft drinks or the odd glass of skimmed or semi-skimmed milk as you feel like it. Avoid fizzy drinks as they will fill you up, spoiling your appetite for your meals.

If you feel hungry later in the evening, have another piece of fruit or some nuts or seeds or, to help you sleep, have a milky drink or a herbal tea.

The great thing about the plan is that you don't have to make any decisions at all if you don't want to – you can follow the programme exactly as it is written. However, if you don't like one of the items on the day's plan (or just feel like changing things), you can choose something similar from another day. So, for example, you may substitute any breakfast with another, any main meal with another – or any whole day with another. You can also have the main meal at lunchtime rather than the evening if that suits you better too. And if you like a particular day's meals, have them every day.

Any piece of fruit is interchangeable with another. I use salads a lot because they are less hassle than preparing vegetables, but if you are not a fan of salad, have a cooked green vegetable instead. The important thing is to make sure you have plenty of fresh, frozen or canned fruit and vegetables every day. Try to include some greens most days and do eat the nuts and seeds too.

Day 1

7–8 am	Get up, make a cup of decaffeinated tea or coffee, have a wash and get dressed (you can dress after breakfast if you prefer).
8–9 am	Prepare and eat your breakfast. **A glass of pure fruit juice** **A bowl of wholegrain cereal with milk and a handful of raisins** **A slice of wholemeal toast with a little butter or low-fat spread and marmalade**
9–11 am	Clear up breakfast. Have a shower and dress, if you have not already done so. Set yourself a task to do now – like clearing up your room. Set some tasks for later and write them on post-it notes to stick around as reminders.
11 am–12 noon	Aerobic exercise: walk, jog, cycle or swim for 15 minutes (see Chapter 10). Freshen up.
12 noon–1 pm	Prepare and eat your lunch. **Roast beef and salad sandwich** (see recipe box) **A fruit yoghurt**

Roast beef and salad sandwich
Spread two slices of wholemeal bread with a little butter or low-fat spread. Top one with sliced roast beef, sliced tomato, slices of cucumber and some lettuce.

Spread the other with a little mayonnaise and a little English mustard and/or horseradish sauce. Sandwich together.

1–2 pm	Clear up lunch. Have a power nap for 20 minutes, if you are tired. If not, read the newspaper or a book, or put on some relaxing music and sit comfortably and listen to it rather than just having it on in the background.
2–4 pm	Do another small task or visit or entertain a friend.

4 pm	Have a snack. **An apple**
4–6 pm	Read a book or other relaxing task.
6–7 pm	Prepare and eat your supper. **Chicken chow mein with plain boiled rice** (ready meal) **Canned pineapple in natural juice with a spoonful of crème fraîche or plain yoghurt**
7 pm–bedtime	Relax: watch TV or a DVD, read a book, do a crossword, etc. Follow the suggestions on 'How to Get a Good Night's Sleep' (see page 32).

Day 2

7–8 am	Get up, make a cup of decaffeinated tea or coffee, have a wash and get dressed (you can dress after breakfast if you prefer).
8–9 am	Prepare and eat your breakfast. **A glass of pure fruit juice** **A bowl of porridge or instant oat cereal with milk and a handful of dried blueberries or cranberries** **A slice of wholemeal toast with a little butter or low-fat spread and Marmite or other yeast extract**
9–11 am	Clear up breakfast. Have a shower and dress, if not already done. Choose a task to do now. Set some tasks for later and write them on post-it notes to stick around as reminders.
11 am–12 noon	Light exercise. Go for a gentle, not brisk, walk or do some other light exercise like some gardening. Freshen up.
12 noon–1 pm	Prepare and eat your lunch. **Tuna and salad wrap** (see recipe box) **A pear**

Tuna and salad wrap
Spread a flour tortilla with mayonnaise and then a little chilli relish. Add some sliced cucumber, sliced onion, if liked, and shredded lettuce.
    Top with a drained, small can of tuna, then roll up.

1–2 pm	Clear up lunch. Have a power nap for 20 minutes, if tired. If not, read the newspaper or a book.
2–4 pm	Do another small task or visit or entertain a friend.
4 pm	Have a snack. **A handful of pumpkin seeds**
4–6 pm	Read a book or other relaxing task.

6–7 pm	Prepare and eat your supper.
	Spinach and ricotta cannelloni (ready meal)
	Sliced tomatoes, topped with slices of onion and French dressing
	A hazelnut (filbert) yoghurt with a handful of grapes
7 pm–bedtime	Relax: watch TV or a DVD, read a book, do a crossword, etc. Follow the suggestions on 'How to Get a Good Night's Sleep' (see page 32).

Day 3

7–8 am	Get up, make a cup of decaffeinated tea or coffee, have a wash and get dressed (you can dress after breakfast if you prefer).
8–9 am	Prepare and eat your breakfast. **A glass of pure fruit juice** **A small can of prunes in natural juice or breakfast compôte with a good spoonful of plain yoghurt, a tablespoon of wheatgerm and a handful of sunflower seeds** **A slice of wholemeal toast, with a little peanut butter**
9–11 am	Clear up breakfast. Have a shower and dress, if not already done. Choose a task to do now. Set some tasks for later and write them on post-it notes to stick around as reminders.
11 am–12 noon	Light exercise. Go for a gentle, not brisk, walk or do some other light exercise like some gardening. Freshen up.
12 noon–1 pm	Prepare and eat your lunch. **Soya bean salad (see recipe box)** **A rye or other wholegrain crispbread**

Soya bean salad
Drain and rinse a small can of soya beans. Put in a bowl with a few cubes of Cheddar cheese, half a chopped green or red (bell) pepper, a slice of onion, chopped, a piece of cucumber, cut into chunks, and a tomato, cut into chunks.

Trickle about a tablespoon of olive oil and a teaspoon of balsamic vinegar over the salad. Add a good grinding of black pepper and a pinch of dried oregano and mix gently.

1–2 pm	Clear up lunch. Have a power nap for 20 minutes, if tired. If not, read the newspaper or a book.
2–4 pm	Do another small task or visit or entertain a friend.

4 pm	Have a snack. **An orange or two satsumas or clementines**
4–6 pm	Read a book or other relaxing task.
6–7 pm	Prepare and eat your supper. **Vegetable-topped pizza** (ready meal) **A bowl of lettuce, topped with a spoonful of coleslaw** **Fresh or thawed frozen raspberries with a raspberry-flavoured fromage frais**
7 pm–bedtime	Relax: watch TV or a DVD, read a book, do a crossword, etc. Follow the suggestions on 'How to Get a Good Night's Sleep' (see page 32).

Day 4

7–8 am	Get up, make a cup of decaffeinated tea or coffee, have a wash and get dressed (you can dress after breakfast if you prefer).
8–9 am	Prepare and eat your breakfast. **A glass of pure fruit juice** **One or two boiled eggs with two slices of wholemeal toast and a little butter or low-fat spread, one with marmalade**
9–11 am	Clear up breakfast. Have a shower and dress, if not already done. Choose a task to do now. Set some tasks for later and write them on post-it notes to stick around as reminders.
11 am–12 noon	Exercise. Do a 20-minute toning or resistance/weight training routine, for upper body if using weights (see page 107 or 117). Freshen up.
12 noon–1 pm	Prepare and eat your lunch. **Fresh vacuum-packed or canned liver pâté** **Wholemeal toast** **Coleslaw and a side salad** **A banana**
1–2 pm	Clear up lunch. Have a power nap for 20 minutes, if tired. If not, read the newspaper or a book.
2–4 pm	Do another small task or visit or entertain a friend.
4 pm	Have a snack. **A handful of pumpkin seeds and raisins**
4–6 pm	Read a book or other relaxing task.
6–7 pm	Prepare and eat your supper. **Thai red or green curry with jasmine rice** (ready meal) **A side salad, sprinkled with soy sauce and lemon juice** **A fruit-flavoured fromage frais with some fresh fruit**
7 pm–bedtime	Relax: watch TV or a DVD, read a book, do a crossword, etc. Follow the suggestions on 'How to Get a Good Night's Sleep' (see page 32).

Day 5

7–8 am	Get up, make a cup of decaffeinated tea or coffee, have a wash and get dressed (you can dress after breakfast if you prefer).
8–9 am	Prepare and eat your breakfast. **A glass of pure fruit juice** **A bowl of muesli with milk** **A slice of wholemeal toast with a little butter or low-fat spread and marmalade**
9–11 am	Clear up breakfast. Have a shower and dress, if not already done. Choose a task to do now. Set some tasks for later and write them on post-it notes to stick around as reminders.
11 am–12 noon	Light exercise. Go for a gentle, not brisk, walk or do some other light exercise like some gardening. Freshen up.
12 noon–1 pm	Prepare and eat your lunch. **Quick cheese and mushroom omelette** (see recipe box) **A sliced tomato** **An apple and two squares (no more) of good-quality chocolate with 70 per cent cocoa solids**

Quick cheese and mushroom omelette

Break two eggs into a bowl. Add two tablespoons of water and a sprinkling of salt and pepper and beat with a fork or whisk until evenly yellow.

Heat a knob of butter or low-fat spread in an omelette pan. Add the egg mixture. Lift and stir gently until the mixture is half set but still runny on top.

Drain a small can of sliced mushrooms and scatter over the omelette. Sprinkle over a small handful of grated cheese. Cover with a lid or foil and continue to heat fairly gently until the mushrooms are hot and the cheese has melted.

1–2 pm	Clear up lunch. Have a power nap for 20 minutes, if tired. If not, read the newspaper or a book.

2–4 pm	Do another small task or visit or entertain a friend.
4 pm	Have a snack. **Two dried apricots and a few whole almonds**
4–6 pm	Read a book or other relaxing task.
6–7 pm	Prepare and eat your supper. **Char-grilled chicken Caesar salad** (see recipe box) **A tomato, cut into quarters or slices** **Canned rice pudding or a pear**

Char-grilled chicken Caesar salad
Cook a frozen char-grilled chicken breast according to the packet instructions (I do it in the microwave).

Tip the lettuce from a small bag of ready-prepared Caesar salad into a bowl, add the croûtons, Parmesan and then the dressing. Toss gently to mix. Slice the chicken breast and put on top.

---

7 pm–bedtime	Relax: watch TV or a DVD, read a book, do a crossword, etc. Follow the suggestions on 'How to Get a Good Night's Sleep' (see page 32).

Day 6

7–8 am	Get up, make a cup of decaffeinated tea or coffee, have a wash and get dressed (you can dress after breakfast if you prefer).
8–9 am	Prepare and eat your breakfast. **A glass of pure fruit juice** **A bowl of wholegrain cereal with milk and a small sliced banana**
9–11 am	Clear up breakfast. Have a shower and dress, if not already done. Choose a task to do now. Set some tasks for later and write them on post-it notes to stick around as reminders.
11 am–12 noon	Light exercise. Go for a gentle, not brisk, walk or do some other light exercise like some gardening. Freshen up.
12 noon–1 pm	Prepare and eat your lunch. **A halved, toasted bagel, topped with soft cheese and a drained can of sardines, mashed with a dash of lemon juice and pepper** **An orange or two satsumas or clementines**
1–2 pm	Clear up lunch. Have a power nap for 20 minutes, if tired. If not, read the newspaper or a book.
2–4 pm	Do another small task or visit or entertain a friend.
4 pm	Have a snack. **A handful of sunflower seeds and sultanas (golden raisins)**
4–6 pm	Read a book or other relaxing task.

6–7 pm	Prepare and eat your supper.
	Two or three grilled (broiled) extra-lean pork sausages
	Instant mash, flavoured with a handful of grated Cheddar cheese and a knob of butter or low-fat spread
	Cooked canned or frozen peas and carrots
	Canned apricots in natural juice and a scoop of ice cream
7 pm–bedtime	Relax: watch TV or a DVD, read a book, do a crossword, etc. Follow the suggestions on 'How to Get a Good Night's Sleep' (see page 32).

Day 7

7–8 am	Get up, make a cup of decaffeinated tea or coffee, have a wash and get dressed (you can dress after breakfast if you prefer).
8–9 am	Prepare and eat your breakfast. **A glass of pure fruit juice** **One or two Weetabix with milk and a handful of chopped dates and a tablespoon of desiccated (shredded) coconut**
9–11 am	Clear up breakfast. Have a shower and dress, if not already done. Choose a task to do now. Set some tasks for later and write them on post-it notes to stick around as reminders.
11 am–12 noon	Light exercise. Go for a gentle, not brisk, walk or do some other light exercise like some gardening. Freshen up.
12 noon–1 pm	Prepare and eat your lunch. **Prawn and mayo sandwich** (see recipe box) **An apple and two squares (no more) of good-quality chocolate with 70 per cent cocoa solids**

Prawn and mayo sandwich
Spread two slices of granary bread with a little butter or low-fat spread. Add mayonnaise to one and top the other with a handful of thawed frozen prawns (shrimp). Add a grinding of black pepper and a layer of watercress or lettuce. Top with the mayo-spread slice and cut in half.

Note: If you forgot to thaw the prawns earlier, put them in cold (**not hot**) water for a few minutes, then drain on kitchen paper (paper towels).

1–2 pm	Clear up lunch. Have a power nap for 20 minutes, if tired. If not, read the newspaper or a book.
2–4 pm	Do another small task or visit or entertain a friend.

4 pm	Have a snack. **A fruit and nut cereal bar or a handful of peanuts or mixed nuts and raisins**
4–6 pm	Read a book or other relaxing task.
6–7 pm	Prepare and eat your supper. **Lasagne** (ready meal) **A salad of rocket, lettuce, tomato, cucumber, red or green (bell) pepper and a few olives, with French dressing** **A slice of orange-fleshed melon with a sprinkling of ground ginger (optional)**
7 pm–bedtime	Relax: watch TV or a DVD, read a book, do a crossword, etc. Follow the suggestions on 'How to Get a Good Night's Sleep' (see page 32).

Day 8

7–8 am	Get up, make a cup of decaffeinated tea or coffee, have a wash and get dressed (you can dress after breakfast if you prefer).
8–9 am	Prepare and eat your breakfast. **A glass of pure fruit juice** **A bowl of porridge or instant hot oat cereal made with milk and a teaspoonful of clear honey** **A slice of wholemeal toast with a little peanut or cashew nut butter**
9–11 am	Clear up breakfast. Have a shower and dress, if not already done. Choose a task to do now. Set some tasks for later and write them on post-it notes to stick around as reminders.
11 am–12 noon	Aerobic exercise. Walk, jog, cycle or swim for 15 minutes (see Chapter 10). Freshen up.
12 noon–1 pm	Prepare and eat your lunch. **Chilli bean and salad wrap** (see recipe box) **A pear**

Chilli bean and salad wrap

Mash a small can of red kidney beans with a splash of hot chilli sauce, to taste. Smear on a flour tortilla and top with some shredded lettuce, chopped cucumber and tomato and a spoonful of plain yoghurt or crème fraîche. Roll up.

1–2 pm	Clear up lunch. Have a power nap for 20 minutes, if tired. If not, read the newspaper or a book.
2–4 pm	Do another small task or visit or entertain a friend.
4 pm	Have a snack. **A fruit and nut cereal bar or a handful of pumpkin seeds**
4–6 pm	Read a book or other relaxing task.

6–7 pm   Prepare and eat your supper.
Steamed salmon with vegetables (ready meal)
A small piece of cheese and an oatcake
A bunch of grapes

7 pm–bedtime   Relax: watch TV or a DVD, read a book, do a
crossword, etc. Follow the suggestions on 'How to
Get a Good Night's Sleep' (see page 32).

Day 9

7–8 am	Get up, make a cup of decaffeinated tea or coffee, have a wash and get dressed (or dress after breakfast if you prefer).
8–9 am	Prepare and eat your breakfast. **A glass of pure fruit juice** **A bowl of muesli with milk** **A slice of wholemeal toast with a little marmalade**
9–11 am	Clear up breakfast. Have a shower and dress, if not already done. Choose a task to do now. Set some tasks for later and write them on post-it notes.
11 am–12 noon	Light exercise. Go for a gentle, not brisk, walk or do some other light exercise like some gardening. Freshen up.
12 noon–1 pm	Prepare and eat your lunch. **A can of minestrone soup, topped with a handful of grated cheese** **A wholegrain bread roll with a little butter or low-fat spread** **A peach or nectarine**
1–2 pm	Clear up lunch. Have a power nap for 20 minutes, if tired. If not, read the newspaper or a book.
2–4 pm	Do another small task or visit or entertain a friend.
4 pm	Have a snack. **A handful of tropical fruit and nut mix**
4–6 pm	Read a book or choose other relaxing task.
6–7 pm	Prepare and eat your supper. **Quiche (ready meal)** **A mixed salad and French dressing or a spoonful of mayonnaise** **A microwaved jacket-baked potato or some boiled fresh or canned baby new potatoes** **A fruit yoghurt with a tablespoon of wheatgerm**
7 pm–bedtime	Relax: watch TV or a DVD, read a book, do a crossword, etc. Follow the suggestions on 'How to Get a Good Night's Sleep' (see page 32).

Day 10

7–8 am	Get up, make a cup of decaffeinated tea or coffee, have a wash and get dressed (you can dress after breakfast if you prefer).
8–9 am	Prepare and eat your breakfast. **A glass of pure fruit juice** **A large ripe banana, whizzed in a blender with two tablespoons of instant oat cereal or wheatgerm, 150 ml/¼ pt milk and a small carton of plain or fruit yoghurt until thick and smooth** **A slice of wholemeal toast, a little butter or low-fat spread and Marmite or other yeast extract**
9–11 am	Clear up breakfast. Have a shower and dress, if not already done. Choose a task to do now. Set some tasks for later and write them on post-it notes to stick around as reminders.
11 am–12 noon	Aerobic exercise. Walk, jog, cycle or swim for 15 minutes (see Chapter 10). Freshen up.
12 noon–1 pm	Prepare and eat your lunch. **One or two sesame-seed pitta breads, filled with hummus, shredded lettuce, sliced cucumber and some sliced black olives** **A kiwi fruit**
1–2 pm	Clear up lunch. Have a power nap for 20 minutes, if tired. If not, read the newspaper or a book.
2–4 pm	Do another small task or visit or entertain a friend.
4 pm	Have a snack. **Two dried figs and a few whole almonds**
4–6 pm	Read a book or other relaxing task.

6–7 pm   Prepare and eat your supper.
Mushroom risotto (see recipe box)
A rocket and tomato salad with a little French dressing
A fruit yoghurt

Mushroom risotto

Empty half a 250 g/9 oz packet of instant mushroom risotto into a pan. Add 300 ml/½ pt/1¼ cups of water and a handful (or a small, drained can) of sliced button mushrooms. Bring to the boil and simmer for 12 minutes.

When cooked, turn into a shallow bowl, top with a drizzle of olive oil and good handful of grated Parmesan.

---

7 pm–bedtime   Relax: watch TV or a DVD, read a book, do a crossword, etc. Follow the suggestions on 'How to Get a Good Night's Sleep' (see page 32).

Day 11

7–8 am	Get up, make a cup of decaffeinated tea or coffee, have a wash and get dressed (you can dress after breakfast if you prefer).
8–9 am	Prepare and eat your breakfast. **A glass of pure fruit juice** **A bowl of wholegrain cereal with milk and a handful of dried cranberries** **A rye crispbread with a little butter or low-fat spread and marmalade**
9–11 am	Clear up breakfast. Have a shower and dress, if not already done. Choose a task to do now. Set some tasks for later and write them on post-it notes to stick around as reminders.
11 am–12 noon	Light exercise. Go for a gentle, not brisk, walk or do some other light exercise like some gardening. Freshen up.
12 noon–1 pm	Prepare and eat your lunch. **Cheese on toast with baked beans** **An apple and two squares (no more) of good-quality chocolate with 70 per cent cocoa solids**
1–2 pm	Clear up lunch. Have a power nap for 20 minutes, if tired. If not, read the newspaper or a book.
2–4 pm	Do another small task or visit or entertain a friend.
4 pm	Have a snack. **A bunch of grapes**
4–6 pm	Read a book or other relaxing task.

6–7 pm   Prepare and eat your supper.
Quick-cook salmon and broccoli pasta
(see recipe box)
A plain yoghurt with a teaspoon of honey

Quick-cook salmon and broccoli pasta
Bring a pan of water to the boil with a pinch of salt. Add a large handful of quick-cook pasta and bring back to the boil. Add a small head of broccoli, cut into small florets. Boil for 4–5 minutes until pasta and broccoli are tender. Drain and tip back in the pan.

Add half a small can of pink salmon, including the bones and juice, and half a small carton of crème fraîche, a pinch of dried oregano and a sprinkling of salt and pepper. Heat through stirring, then tip into a bowl to serve.

Note: Keep the remainder of the salmon in the fridge for tomorrow's supper.

---

7 pm–bedtime   Relax: watch TV or a DVD, read a book, do a crossword, etc. Follow the suggestions on 'How to Get a Good Night's Sleep' (see page 32).

Day 12

7–8 am	Get up, make a cup of decaffeinated tea or coffee, have a wash and get dressed (dress after breakfast if you prefer).
8–9 am	Prepare and eat your breakfast. **A glass of pure fruit juice** **One or two boiled eggs and a slice of wholemeal toast with a little butter or low-fat spread and a little Marmite**
9–11 am	Clear up breakfast. Have a shower and dress, if not already done. Choose a task to do now. Set some tasks for later and write them on post-it notes to stick around as reminders.
11 am–12 noon	Exercise. Do a 20-minute toning or resistance/weight training routine, for lower body if using weights (see page 107 or 117). Freshen up.
12 noon–1 pm	Prepare and eat your lunch. **Salmon and cucumber wrap** (see recipe box) **Two tomatoes, cut into wedges** **A plain yoghurt with a handful of raisins**

Salmon and cucumber wrap
Mix the rest of the salmon from last night with a tablespoon of mayonnaise. Spread on a flour tortilla and top with thin slices of cucumber. Fold in half, then half again to form a cone.

1–2 pm	Clear up lunch. Have a power nap for 20 minutes, if tired. If not, read the newspaper or a book.
2–4 pm	Do another small task or visit or entertain a friend.
4 pm	Have a snack. **An oatcake with a little peanut butter**
4–6 pm	Read a book or other relaxing task.

6–7 pm   Prepare and eat your supper.
Tandoori chicken with a vegetable curry (ready meal)
A side salad and a wedge of lemon, to squeeze over
An orange or two satsumas or clementines

7 pm–bedtime   Relax: watch TV or a DVD, read a book, do a crossword, etc. Follow the suggestions on 'How to Get a Good Night's Sleep' (see page 32).

Day 13

7–8 am	Get up, make a cup of decaffeinated tea or coffee, have a wash and get dressed (you can dress after breakfast if you prefer).
8–9 am	Prepare and eat your breakfast. **A glass of pure fruit juice** **A bowl of wholegrain cereal with milk and a sliced banana**
9–11 am	Clear up breakfast. Have a shower and dress, if not already done. Choose a task to do now. Set some tasks for later and write them on post-it notes to stick around as reminders.
11 am–12 noon	Light exercise. Go for a gentle, not brisk, walk or do some other light exercise like some gardening. Freshen up.
12 noon–1 pm	Prepare and eat your lunch. **One or two granary rolls, filled with sliced ham, lettuce, sliced tomato and cucumber and a little mayonnaise and English mustard** **An apple and two squares (no more) of good-quality chocolate with 70 per cent cocoa solids**
1–2 pm	Clear up lunch. Have a power nap for 20 minutes, if tired. If not, read the newspaper or a book.
2–4 pm	Do another small task or visit or entertain a friend.
4 pm	Have a snack. **A handful of peanuts or mixed nuts and raisins**
4–6 pm	Read a book or other relaxing task. Prepare your evening snack.
6–7 pm	Prepare and eat your supper. **Chicken, lamb or beef and vegetable stew or casserole** (fresh or frozen ready meal) **Fresh or frozen broccoli** **A plain yoghurt with a teaspoon of clear honey**
7 pm–bedtime	Relax: watch TV or a DVD, read a book, do a crossword, etc. Follow the suggestions on 'How to Get a Good Night's Sleep' (see page 32).

Day 14

7–8 am	Get up, make a cup of decaffeinated tea or coffee, have a wash and get dressed (you can dress after breakfast if you prefer).
8–9 am	Prepare and eat your breakfast. **A glass of pure fruit juice** **A bowl of porridge or hot instant oat cereal with milk and a teaspoon of honey** **A slice of wholemeal toast with a little butter or low-fat spread and marmalade**
9–11 am	Clear up breakfast. Have a shower and dress, if not already done. Choose a task to do now. Set some tasks for later and write them on post-it notes to stick around as reminders.
11 am–12 noon	Light exercise. Go for a gentle, not brisk, walk or do some other light exercise like some gardening. Freshen up.
12 noon–1 pm	Prepare and eat your lunch. **A small can of pilchards in tomato sauce** **Quick Russian salad** (see recipe box) **A kiwi fruit**

Quick Russian salad
Drain a small can of diced mixed vegetables and mix with a tablespoon of mayonnaise, a good grinding of black pepper and a handful of sesame seeds.

1–2 pm	Clear up lunch. Have a power nap for 20 minutes, if tired. If not, read the newspaper or a book.
2–4 pm	Do another small task or visit or entertain a friend.
4 pm	Have a snack. **A teacake, either plain or toasted, with a little butter or low-fat spread**
4–6 pm	Read a book or other relaxing task.

6–7 pm   Prepare and eat your supper.
                   Lamb tagine with couscous (ready meal)
                   Fresh, frozen or canned green beans

7 pm–bedtime   Relax: watch TV or a DVD, read a book, do a
                   crossword, etc. Follow the suggestions on 'How to
                   Get a Good Night's Sleep' (see page 32).

More quick and easy ideas for main meals

Vegetable pasta with Parmesan: Cook a large handful of quick-cook pasta, with a diced (bell) pepper added to the water for the last 2 minutes. Drain, then mix with a roasted vegetable stir-in sauce. Return to pan and heat through. Top with grated Parmesan and serve with a large salad.

Creamy mushroom-topped pork, beef or lamb with rice and vegetables: Grill (broil) a chop or steak. Heat a small can of creamed mushrooms as a sauce. Serve with microwaved or boil-in-the-bag rice, canned or fresh carrots and fresh or frozen broccoli or shredded cabbage.

Salmon with cheesy mash and vegetables: Grill (broil) or poach a salmon steak. Serve on a bed of instant (or freshly cooked) mashed potato, flavoured with grated cheese, with peas and canned or cooked fresh tomatoes.

Instant paella: Cook a small packet of savoury vegetable rice, according to the packet instructions, with a diced raw chicken breast and a couple of sliced mushrooms added at the start. Add a good handful of frozen prawns and a pinch of dried oregano for the last 3 minutes' cooking time. Serve with a salad.

Italian-style stuffed pasta: Cook a portion of dried stuffed spinach and ricotta tortellini according to the packet directions, then drain. Mix with a tomato and Mascarpone stir-in sauce and heat through. Top with grated cheese and serve with a mixed salad.

Tuna Mornay: Mix a small can of tuna, drained and flaked, with a small can of diced mixed vegetables in a small flameproof dish. Whisk an egg with a small carton of low-fat crème fraîche, a generous handful of grated Cheddar cheese, a good pinch of dried mixed herbs and some salt and pepper. Spread over the tuna, then grill (broil) until bubbling, golden and just set. Serve with a green salad.

Grilled gammon/ham steak with cheese and tomato: Grill (broil) a gammon or ham steak on one side for 2–3 minutes. Turn over and spread the other side with a little grainy mustard, then add a sliced tomato, a sprinkling of dried basil and some slices of Cheddar cheese. Grill until bubbling and the cheese has melted. Serve with grilled frozen rosti and some fresh, frozen or canned green beans.

Maintaining your diet

Once you have established good exercise and eating habits and are enjoying your food again, you may find you are ready to do a little more cooking for yourself. You can continue to follow the diet plan, mixing and matching meals and menus as you like, but also start to include the quick main-meal ideas on page 95 and the healthy ready-meal options suggested in the list on page 28. Remember to add extra fresh vegetables or salad to them for the added goodness.

Then, when you are ready, you can sample the easy recipes at the end of the book. These, along with your continued exercise programme, will go on helping you to keep your body and mind fit and active.

chapter ten

All about Exercise

Exercise is important for everyone and for people who are depressed it can be a real morale-booster. You don't have to embark immediately on a strenuous daily work-out, although it's a good idea to do something active every day. The sessions built into the eating plans are very simple and scheduled only twice a week to start with, and even when you are well into the exercise regime, there are lots of rest days.

This programme is meant as a guide only. All of the following exercise suggestions can be done without joining a gym or special club. Apart from saving money and transport costs, it does mean you can start your routine without having to interact with anyone if you aren't up to it. However, joining some kind of group is very helpful as part of your recovery and to keep you motivated. So, as and when you feel ready, it might be a good idea to do just that.

As with any new exercise regime, you should check with your doctor or specialist before beginning it.

Watchpoints

- If you're new to exercise, start slowly. It is best to do just enough than to work too hard. Rest is important, too, so I've started you off with just two sessions in the first week, combined with light exercise on other days.

- If at any time you feel dizzy or sick or notice any discomfort, then stop exercising.

- The exercises should make you feel slightly tired but will eventually give you more energy as well as toning you up and giving you that feel-good factor.

● You must eat properly if you are going to exercise regularly or you won't have enough energy to enjoy it. So follow the diet plan on either page 39 or page 68. If you choose not to (though I recommend you do), then make sure you eat plenty of nutritious foods – see page 24.

Warming up and cooling down

These are both are very important. If you don't warm up properly before embarking on any sort of strenuous exercise, you risk injuring yourself; and a period of cooling-down will help you to stretch your muscles so that you don't ache too much the next day. So make sure you follow this advice before and after every exercise routine.

Your warm-up prepares your muscles for exercise by raising your heartbeat and breathing rates whilst increasing your body temperature and preventing injury. It should consist of gradually increasing the exercise intensity, thus raising your breathing rate, for about 5–10 minutes. Marching on the spot, swinging the arms, jogging on the spot and so on are all good ways to warm up.

Cooling down should do the opposite – you should gradually reduce the intensity of the exercise so that your breathing rate drops over a period of 5–10 minutes. So do the same jogging and swinging the arms, but gradually slow it down until your heart is no longer pumping fast. Do some stretches too (see below).

Stretches

Stretches should each be held for 30 seconds and should include (see pictures):

● Shoulders

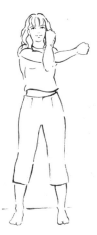

- Chest

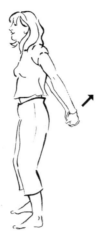

- Back of arms

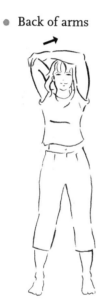

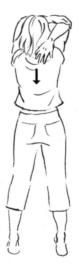

- Back

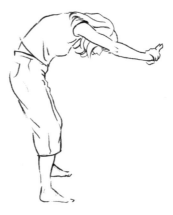

- Stomach

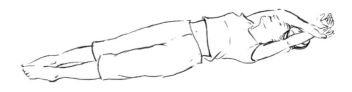

- Thighs

- Calves and backs of thighs

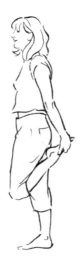

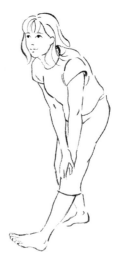

Aerobic exercise

Aerobic exercise should make your heart beat faster, make you feel warmer and breathe more quickly. You are not aiming to make yourself feel exhausted, sweating and gasping for breath! Remember the last time you ran for the bus? That's the feeling you are aiming for and you should try to keep it up for at least 15 minutes. The more regularly you do it, the fitter you will become.

Here are suggestions of what to do, how, when and where. I have started with walking – it's easy, doesn't need any special equipment and it's free! – but instead of walking, you could go jogging, cycling or swimming. You could also join an aerobics or dance class, which would also help you interact with people when you feel ready.

Walking
Benefits include

- Can be done anytime, anywhere.

- Is easy to do, needing minimal equipment and no training.

- Provides low-impact exercise, minimising risk of injury.

- Can improve physical fitness as well as mental wellbeing if done regularly and for long enough.

- Can be done while listening to music, which makes it even more enjoyable.

Equipment needed

- **Good shoes:** Walking shoes should be supportive and have either a small heel or no heel at all. They should be well-fitting and flexible. Note that walking and running shoes are different so if you're thinking of buying a new pair, you should make sure you state what you want them for: this may be only walking or both walking and jogging if you're thinking of progressing to jogging later on.

- **Comfortable clothing:** Go for loose-fitting and quick-drying clothing allowing freedom of motion and efficient 'sweat-removal'.

Good technique

It is important to 'walk tall'. Don't panic if this sounds complicated, most people walk like this anyway!

- Relax your upper body, expand your chest, be conscious of your stomach muscles – hold them in to support your spine and pelvis – and keep your head and chin up.

- Let your arms swing freely and naturally.

Handy hints

- Walk whenever possible. For example, take the stairs instead of a lift (elevator) or escalator and, preferably, walk to the shops instead of taking the car. If taking the bus, get off a stop early and walk the last bit. If you're travelling by train and the station is near enough, walk to it instead of taking the car.

- Walk at a good pace and with a purpose. Don't just stroll along idly. Imagine you are trying to keep up with someone in front of you. The more you put into your walk, the better you'll feel.

- Safety first. Walk only in well-lit, public areas and always let someone know where you're going and what time you'll be back. Take a mobile phone and some money with you and walk with someone else if possible.

Jogging

Benefits include

- Can be done anytime, anywhere.

- Is easy to do, needing minimal equipment and minimal training.

- Provides excellent aerobic exercise (heart and lungs).

- Fitness and mental benefits can be seen relatively quickly.

Equipment needed

- **Good shoes:** These needn't be expensive but must fit correctly and allow good support, shock-absorption and flexibility. Your local sports shop should be able to advise you but remember that the most expensive trainers are not necessarily the best ones.

- Comfortable clothing: Your clothes should allow easy movement and dry quickly. Breathable fabrics are best of all.

Good technique

- Do what comes naturally – everyone has their own individual jogging style. Enjoy it!

- Try and relax your upper body, keeping your shoulders down. This should be less tiring. If you tense up, you'll feel your body starting to protest.

- Once you've been doing it for a while, think about your posture a bit more. Keep your head up and look straight in front of you (this will stop you leaning too far forwards).

Handy hints

- Don't bounce too much – this wastes your energy.

- Jog relaxed, jog tall and enjoy.

- Be aware of any 'niggles' that may indicate that you need to rest. If your body complains, don't ignore it or you'll simply make things worse.

- If you begin to feel out of breath, shorten your stride but don't stop. You'll find you begin to feel better.

- Safety first. Always jog in public places that are well lit. Take money and a mobile phone and always let people know where you are going and for how long.

Cycling
Benefits include

- Can be as easy or as hard as you like.

- It is an excellent alternative to jogging if you have any knee, ankle or hip problems, as there is no impact on the joints.

- Can be more interesting than jogging or walking as the distance covered is much greater and you may be able to get out in the country or discover some parts of your town or city or cycle paths you didn't know before.

- Burns a relatively large number of calories.

Equipment needed

- A bike – obviously! A mountain bike is a good choice as it can be used both on the road and on rough terrain and tends to be more comfortable. But any old one will do (as long as the brakes work and the tyres are sound).

- A decent helmet is very important.

- Optional extras include: padded cycling shorts (for comfort), glasses to keep grit out of your eyes and some reflective clothing.

Good technique

- Adopt a posture that protects your lower back: relax your upper body, keep your arms loose and bend forward slightly at the waist.

- Try to change your hand position regularly to prevent stiffness and hold the handle bars lightly.

Handy hints

- Maintain a comfortable, regular pedalling speed and change the gears accordingly as you go up/down hill or into the wind.

- Follow the rules of the road and think safety. Make sure you wear clearly visible clothing and use lights as necessary. It is best to cycle in well-lit areas and preferably with someone else. If you have to cycle alone, cycle in well lit areas.

- Take a phone and money with you and always let friends/relatives know where you're going, for how long and when you'll be back.

- Always take water with you (or a water-based drink) and drink regularly before you get thirsty.

- Brake gently!

- Learn how to fix a flat tyre (easy-to follow instructions are available on the internet at www.halfords.com, in their advice section under *how to guides … bikes*)

Swimming

Benefits include

- This is one of the most complete forms of exercise.

- There is no impact on your joints at all.

- Provides a really good aerobic workout that utilises all of the major muscle groups.

- Promotes excellent flexibility.

- Costs very little.

Equipment needed

- A swimsuit

- Optional extras: goggles, float (if you want to work the upper and lower body separately or if you aren't that confident a swimmer), swimming hat

- Somewhere to swim – this is most likely to be your local pool, but you could also go to a swimming lake or the sea (preferably manned by lifeguards).

Good technique

Choose the stroke that you prefer and work on it. The fastest stroke is front crawl. To perfect this, try these top tips.

- Keep the strokes long by reaching forward as far as possible and pulling back all the way to your thigh.

- Keep your elbow as the highest point of your arm to generate maximum power.

- Make your hands enter the water thumb first and as far in front of you as possible.

- Kick up and down from your hips, not your knees. Keep your kicks small, to increase your thrust.

If you prefer breaststroke, which is slower but can be powerful once mastered, try these tips.

- Keep your body level and flat just under the surface of the water.

- Keep your shoulders in line with your hips.

- Work your legs like a frog, drawing them in towards your bottom, then kicking out to the sides and round, to straight legs with feet together. Thrust your arms forward with your hands together as you kick out to the sides, for best propulsion.

- Draw your arms round in a wide circle as you draw your feet up towards your bottom in the frog position, ready to kick and thrust forward again.

- When you become proficient you should be able to 'rock' in the water, rather like a dolphin, lifting your head up to draw breath, then breathing out as you thrust forward with your head going down into the water.

Handy hints

- Never swim alone or shortly after a meal.

- To increase your enjoyment, try using swimming aids.

- When (and if) you feel like it, join a water aerobics class.

Other aerobic options

Of course, any other kind of sport that gets you moving and makes you slightly hot and out of breath is also ideal. So if you like to kick a football around, play badminton or tennis, even play frisbee with your friends, those are all great options. It doesn't matter if you just hit a tennis ball against the garage wall, kick a ball around the garden or the park or play badminton with the children, it's all good exercise. If it's something you like, you don't have to be any good at it – just do it!

Exercises for toning up

As well as aerobic exercise, it is good to do some exercise that tones your body and for this Pilates is a good choice. It comprises a holistic exercise approach to whole-body conditioning, concentrating on strengthening and stabilising deep-lying abdominal muscles. It aims to realign, strengthen and tone the entire body, stabilising and mobilising muscles, enhancing posture and flexibility. Practising Pilates regularly can often eliminate chronic aches and pains.

Benefits include

- Improves flexibility.

- Builds greater muscular strength and tone.

- Lowers stress levels.

- Promotes greater immune efficiency.

- Improves posture.

- Can be done anywhere, at any time.

Equipment needed

- Comfortable clothing.

- A mat – or just the floor!

How to start

Before you begin always warm up (see page 98). Next, you must learn the correct body position, known as the 'neutral spine' position, which is the starting position for all Pilates exercises.

- Lie on your back with your knees slightly bent.

- Place your hands over your lower stomach, thumb ends touching and finger ends pointing towards each other to form a triangle. Rock your pelvis back and forth until your hands are completely parallel with the floor.

- You have now reached your 'neutral spine' position.

● Now you need to contract your deep stomach muscles. The muscular contraction is a very light one and a common mistake is to clench too hard. Clench your pelvic floor muscles (imagine you're stopping yourself in the middle of having a wee). Draw in your belly button towards your spine whilst still breathing in a comfortable, relaxed way. This abdominal movement of contracting your deep abdominal muscles stabilises your lower back and prepares the body for movement.

The next few pages contain 12 simple Pilates exercises. Try just a couple of repeats of each one to start with, then do a few more repetitions each time you do your exercises until you feel stretched but not worn out – the technical description is 'to comfortable fatigue'. If you can't do some of them, don't worry. Either do what you comfortably can, or leave that exercise until you have run through the programme a few times, then try again.

You might like to put on some quiet, relaxing music in the background, but don't use anything with a strong beat, as you might for an aerobics class. It is important that you do all the exercises slowly and calmly, breathing deeply and regularly as you do, and keeping a gentle hold on those tummy muscles while you exercise. You'll soon find you improve steadily.

While you are exercising, your breathing rhythm is important. Breathe in deeply from your rib cage before you start, then breathe out as you carry out the movement, pulling your rib cage in.

Most important of all, try to concentrate only on your body – don't think about anything else except your breathing and your muscles. This will not only help you do the exercises well, it will really help your mood. Don't forget to cool down (see page 98) when you have finished your routine.

Basic curl up

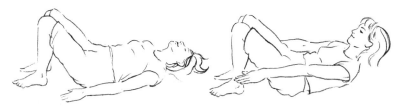

- Keep your neck straight and look at the ceiling, with your arms straight out in front of you, with knees slightly bent and feet flat on the floor.

- Gradually lift your upper body off the floor, bit by bit, and sit up. Just go halfway if you cannot manage sitting right up.

- Gradually curl back down again, keeping the movement slow and even.

The 100

- An advancement of the curl up, with feet either on the floor or raised (which is harder).

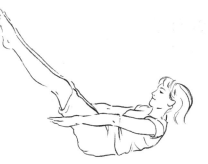

- Hold the position, whilst beating your hands gently on or near the floor as you count, in time with your breathing: 'In, two, three, four, five, out, two, three, four, five, in ...'. The aim is to count to 100, but you should work up to this gradually – start with 20 beats.

Spine curl

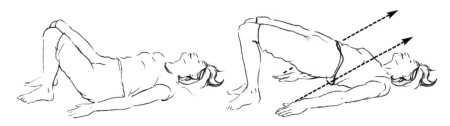

- Lie flat on the floor with your knees bent and feet flat on the floor.

- Gradually 'peel' your spine off the floor from pelvis to shoulder level, then lift your arms until they are level with your eyebrows. You will have to work to keep your balance.

- Gradually curl back down again, feeling your vertebrae touching the floor one at a time.

Advanced spine curl

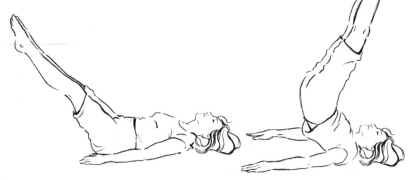

- Keep your arms flat on the floor. Keep your legs straight, feet together.

- Lift your feet up towards your head as far as possible.

- Now press down with your arms to help push your legs further over your head, 'peeling' your spine off the floor as you do so, from pelvis to shoulder level, then move slowly back down to start position.

Leg stretch

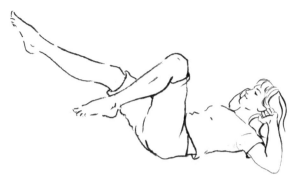

- Lie flat on the floor with your knees slightly bent and feet flat on the floor.

- Gradually 'peel' your spine off the floor from pelvis to shoulder level, and then raise both feet off the floor and straighten one leg to a 45° angle from the floor.

- Alternately straighten your legs with your head and shoulders off the floor.

Table top

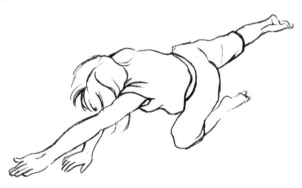

- Kneel down on hands and knees and maintain a neutral spine.

- Whilst looking at the floor, extend your left arm and right leg parallel with the floor. Hold for 5 seconds, then repeat with the opposite arm and leg.

The cat

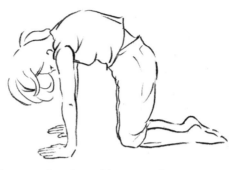

- Kneel down on hands and knees and maintain a neutral spine.

- Looking at the floor, arch your back, hold for 5 seconds and then return to neutral spine.

Thread the needle

- Kneel down on hands and knees and maintain a neutral spine. Take your right hand off the floor and 'thread' it under your left armpit, following through slightly by rotating your trunk and turning your head so you are looking over your shoulder.

- Hold for 5 seconds before doing the same with the other arm.

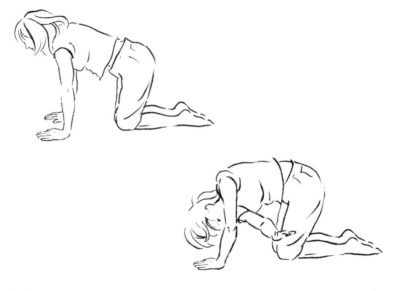

The dog

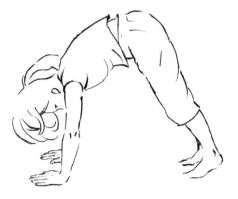

- Stand with your feet slightly apart, then bend down and place your hands on the floor. Raise your hips until your legs are straight with your weight on your toes.

- Gradually lower your heels to the floor whilst breathing out – you will feel tension at the back of your thighs.

- The closer your feet are to your hands the harder it is.

The star

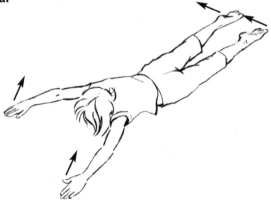

- Lie flat on your stomach, arms and legs stretched out like a star.

- Keeping your arms and legs straight, raise them off the floor. Hold for 5 seconds, then relax.

- To make the exercise more challenging, follow the same instructions but alternately raise one leg and the opposite arm and hold for 5 seconds.

Swimming

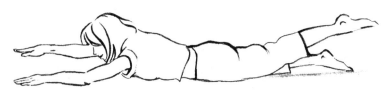

- Lie flat on your stomach with your arms and legs straight, shoulders down and relaxed.
- Stretch and raise your right arm and left leg, keeping your shoulder down, then relax.
- Repeat with your left arm and right leg.

The seal

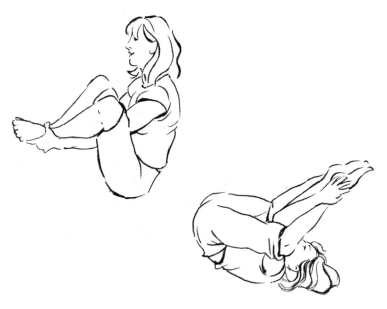

- Sit upright with feet together, off the floor.
- Thread your hands between your legs and hold on to your feet, keeping your legs as straight as possible.
- Rock back gently until your shoulders are on the floor and then rock back to the start, maintaining balance and clapping feet together three times, like a seal.

The chalk circle

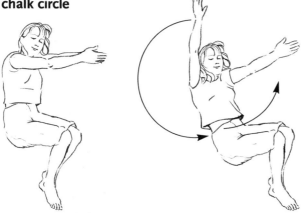

- Lie on your left side with your knees drawn up, arms straight out on the floor with hands together.

- Raise your right arm and draw a circle with your right hand, moving it over your head, behind you, down to your legs and round back to the starting position, following it with your eyes all the time.

- Repeat on the other side.

The side leg raise

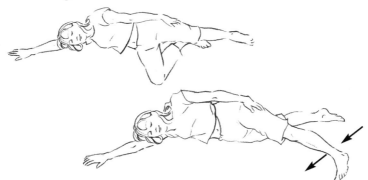

- Lie on your right side with your right leg bent and left hand resting along your left thigh. Keeping your left leg straight, raise it off the floor and, holding it in line with your hip, move it round to the front, to an angle of 90°. Hold for 5 seconds and move back to the start position.

- Repeat on the other side.

Advanced leg raise

- Lie on your side with both legs out straight.

- Raise both legs off the floor and hold for 5 seconds, then relax. Repeat on the other side.

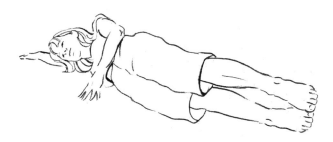

The underlying leg raise

- Lie on your right side with your left leg bent and right leg straight.

- Raise your right (lower) leg off the ground (keeping it straight), hold for 5 seconds, then lower it again and relax. Repeat on the other side.

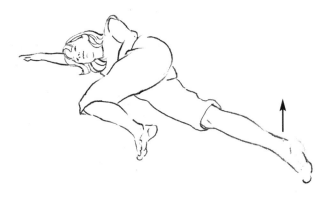

Resistance/weight training

Working with weights is an option you may like to consider when you are further on the road to recovery. It does **not** mean working with heavy weights: it involves slow, regulated bending and stretching, sometimes with light weights to add a little resistance to help build up your muscle strength. But it does require a bit more energy or concentration than you may have right now. If so, just skip this section entirely – you can always come back to it when you feel you are ready. Remember, you are in charge of what you do and don't do, and you need only do things at your own pace. 'Slow and steady' are the key words on your road to recovery.

Weight training can be done in one of three ways:

● At home with make-shift weights

● At home with 'proper weights'

● At a gym.

The at-home options are great when you are using light to moderate weights. The weights should be light enough for you to be able to do three to five sets of 12–15 repetitions for each exercise and you must start using light weights only. If you don't have any proper weights, you can go for the home-made option, using 400–500 g cans of food or 500 ml plastic bottles of water; they are the right weight (around 500 g each) and easy to hold. On pages 120–129 you'll find step-by-step instructions on how to use them to work out safely and effectively.

Later on, you might think about buying some weights from a sports store if you find you are enjoying the exercise and benefiting from it. Start with the lightest, which will be about 1 kg each. You can also buy weights by mail order or over the internet but you should always try out the real thing in a shop first.

You may find this is just your kind of exercise and, when you are feeling more like your old self, you may want to join a gym. Have a taster session or a tour so you can get to know the atmosphere, as well as the facilities, and check the price structure – you don't want to be worrying whether it is too expensive. If you are paying monthly, work out how often you need to go to make it worthwhile; if you are only going once or twice a week, a pay-as-you-go option may be better – check whether this is available. Once you have joined, a programme can be tailor-made for you and supervision and advice is always on hand, so do take advantage of it. An exercise programme designed specifically for you will not only be better for you, it will also be more varied. Going to a gym will also give you the opportunity to meet and chat to more people while you are there.

Benefits include

- Provides a whole-body workout in a relatively short time.
- Can be done at home.
- Will help you to tone muscles, increase endurance and flexibility and burn fat.

Equipment needed

- Supportive shoes with a good grip and a flat heel/sole
- Comfortable, breathable clothing
- Weights
- A mirror
- A supportive hard upright chair.

Handy hints

- Start at an easy level. Ensure the weights you are lifting are really light – you need to learn to do the exercises properly without any strain and using even light weights will still benefit you.
- Always check that the weight in each hand is the same, if you're using two.
- Make sure you are standing on a flat, even surface.
- Stand tall and keep your back straight.
- If you are using a chair, ensure it is hard and supports your back. Try to avoid sitting on a stool as you will then need to concentrate on sitting upright and you will have to work harder to do so.
- Breathe deeply while you work out – don't hold your breath! Breathe in when you rest, and breathe out when you move.
- Do each exercise relatively slowly, counting 'one, two' slowly each way.

● Do a full range of exercises so you work all your major muscles, not just one part of your body.

The workout explained in the next few pages provides a simple, complete, basic exercise programme. It offers you one exercise for each major muscle group that you should work (and occasionally a second option). Look at the illustrations on pages 120–129 to check you are doing the exercises properly.

Start with six repetitions of each exercise, then over a period of weeks gradually work up to 12–15 repetitions.

As you do the exercises, you should feel yourself becoming warmer than usual, perhaps a little out of breath on some exercises, and you should be aware that your muscles are working. Do not strain. If you can only do four repeats, that's fine. Do the whole programme on four repeats for a few sessions, then try five when you are ready. Try not to be too impatient.

Above all, concentrate on what you are doing. Think about your body, feel how it is reacting to the resistance; remember to breathe deeply and slowly, and it will really help to stop your mind racing round your problems.

As I said, you should work out your whole body. Ideally, you should work your upper and lower body at alternate sessions. To help you with this, I have marked the exercises 'U' – for upper – and 'L' – for lower. Keep this in mind if you do the exercises in a different order, or if you substitute others.

Remember, you are working up to 12–15 repeats of each exercise at your own pace.

Chest press
U: for the chest

- **Start position:** Lie on your back on a firm surface, such as a carpet or a mat on the floor. Bend your knees and put your feet flat on the floor. Hold a weight in each hand. Have your elbows bent, palms facing up, fingers towards your head.

- **Movement and end position:** Push up to the ceiling, nice and slowly. Your arms should be straight although with 'soft' elbows (don't fully lock them by making them rigid).

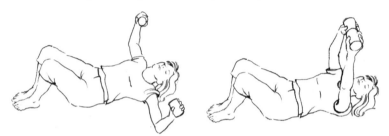

Half press-up
U: for the chest

- **Start position:** Kneel on the floor, with your ankles crossed or parallel, and put your hands a shoulder-width apart with your palms flat on the floor (the further out to the sides, the harder it will be).

- **Movement and end position:** Keep your knees on the ground and bend your arms as far as you can; when you have had plenty of practice, you may be able to bend your arms until your nose touches the floor. Then straighten your arms again to return to the start position.

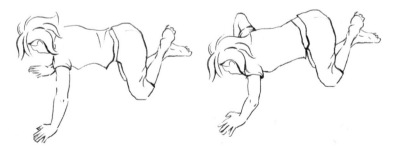

Full press-up

U: for the chest

Note: Don't even try this until you can easily do 15 half press-ups (see page 120).

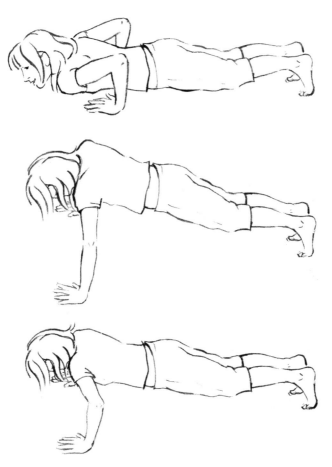

- **Start position:** Lie on your front on a firm surface with your feet together, toes tucked under, palms flat on the floor next to your armpits.

- **Movement and end position:** Push up until your arms are straight, then bend your arms until your nose touches the floor again. The wider apart your arms, the more you are working your chest (rather than your arms).

Upright row
U: for the upper back

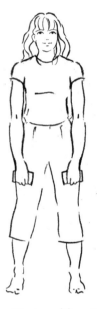 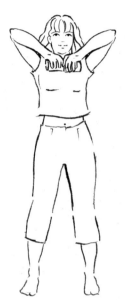

- **Start position:** Stand tall and straight, with a weight in each hand and your knees slightly bent. Your arms should be relaxed in front of you with the weights touching the front of your thighs.

- **Movement and end position:** Keeping the weights in the same line, move them up to under your chin by bending your elbows. Then return to the start position.

Bent-over row
U: for the upper back

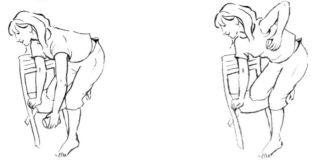

- **Start position:** Stand by a chair. Put your right knee on the seat and support yourself with your right hand also on the seat. Keep your back and neck straight. Hold a weight in your left hand, keeping your arm relaxed and hanging straight.

- **Movement and end position:** Keeping your back and neck still, bend your elbow and move the weight up to your chest, then back down until the arm is straight.

- Turn around and repeat with the other arm.

Shoulder press
U: for the shoulders

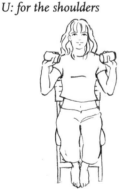
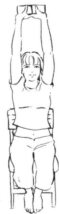

- **Start position:** Sit on a chair with your back supported. Make sure you are sitting up tall and straight. Hold a weight in each hand, resting on your lap. Lift the weights to shoulder height, keeping your palms facing forward.

- **Movement and end position:** Push the weights up to meet above your head, then bring them back down to your shoulders.

Biceps curls

U: for the arms

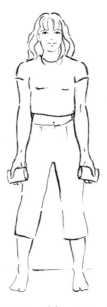 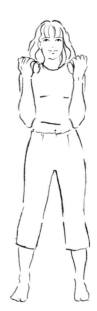

- **Start position:** Stand tall and straight with a weight in each hand, with your arms hanging straight, palms facing forward.

- **Movement and end position:** Bend your elbows until your hands touch your shoulders, then take them back down.

Triceps dips

U: for the arms

This is a more challenging exercise. Bend only a little at first and do just a few repetitions. The important thing is to keep your back straight.

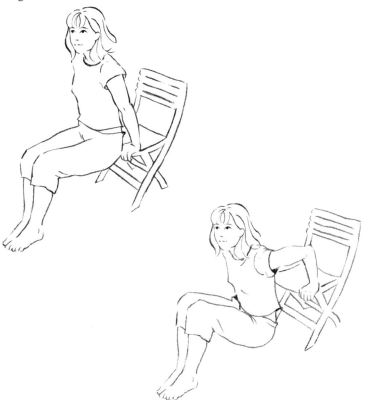

- **Start position:** Sit on the edge of a hard chair with your feet flat on the floor. Place the heel of your hands on the edge of the chair, keeping your arms close to your sides, with your fingers over the edge. Keep your knees bent and raise your bottom off the chair so that you are hovering above the floor. If you allow your feet to move forward, this will make the exercise harder, so keep them below your knees to start with.

- **Movement and end position:** Bend your arms and lower yourself down until your elbows are at right angles and your bottom is above the floor, if you can. Then push through your hands to straighten your arms and return to the start position.

Front crunches

U and L: for the stomach

Start this exercise gently, just lifting slightly off the floor, and doing only a few repetitions. It is important that you use your stomach muscles. If you feel you are straining your neck, stop.

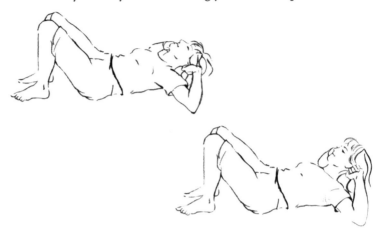

- **Start position:** Lie flat on a hard surface with your knees bent, your hands behind your ears and your neck straight.

- **Movement and end position:** Keeping your neck straight and your chin pointing towards the ceiling, lift your shoulders only off the floor, then lower them back down slowly.

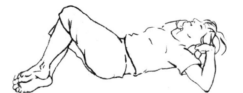

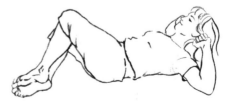

- To exercise the muscles at the sides of your abdomen, do the same exercise with your legs bent to one side (remember to do both sides).

Leg and arm stretch

L: for your lower back and buttocks

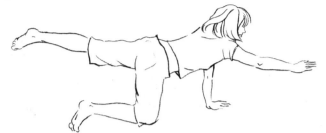

- **Start position:** Get down on your hands and knees with your back straight.

- **Movement and end position:** Raise and straighten the right arm and left leg simultaneously, keeping them in line. Do not allow your back to arch. Pause for a second at maximum stretch, then lower your arm and leg to the starting position and repeat with the opposite limbs.

Squats

L: for your legs and buttocks

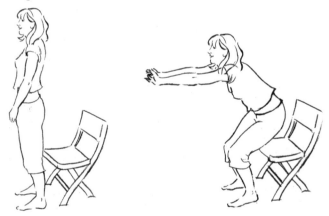

- **Start position:** Stand tall and relaxed in front of a chair with the back of your knees touching the chair.

- **Movement and end position:** Bend your knees as though you were going to sit down and stretch your arms out in front as you do so. Allow your bottom just to touch the chair, then stand up again.

- You can hold weights if you like to make the exercise harder.

Lunges

L: for your legs and buttocks

Don't step too far forward to begin with as you may find it hard to get back. Try a few gentle lunges first to get used to the movement.

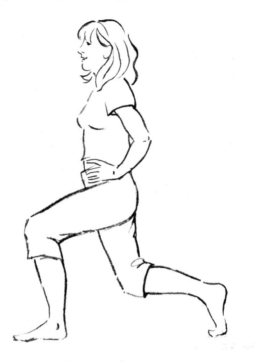

- **Start position:** Stand up straight.

- **Movement and end position:** Take a large step forward, keeping your back straight and bending your front knee to a comfortable angle. Make sure you can always see your toes in front of your front knee. The lower you dip your back knee, the harder the exercise will be. Lift your front foot and step back to the start position, then lunge forward on the other leg.

- You can hold weights if you like to make the exercise harder.

Calf raises

L: for your legs and buttocks

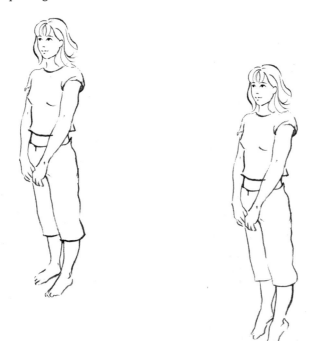

- **Start position:** Stand in a relaxed posture with your feet flat on the floor.

- **Movement and end position:** Raise yourself up on to your toes, then back down on to the floor.

- You can hold weights if you like to make the exercise harder.

chapter eleven

Your Ten-week Exercise Programme

Variety is the spice of life and that goes for exercise too! The greater range of exercises you introduce, the more motivated and interested you will be and the better your body and mind will respond. This programme incorporates both aerobic exercise – such as walking and swimming – and exercise for toning and strength, such as weight training or Pilates.

We have already covered the first two weeks in the two-week diet and exercise plans on pages 39 and 68. These gave you a complete hour-by-hour programme in which you are encouraged simply to go for a walk or take some basic exercise. Now we are going to introduce the remaining eight weeks of the exercise programme in a table that you can follow on a day-to-day basis. Remember to continue to maintain one of the eating plans suggested. Simply follow the days as before, adding in these new exercises at appropriate times of the day. For each week, and each day of the week, I have suggested the type of exercise you should do on that day, and how many minutes you should do it for – it's that simple. On the 'rest' days, continue to do light exercise as before.

Don't be put off by the fact that everything is displayed in a table – this makes it very easy to follow.

What type of exercise

Look at the table on page 131. It starts on Week 3, as Weeks 1 and 2 are included in the meals plans.

Where you see this icon **Ⓐ**, you should choose an aerobic-type exercise, such as walking, jogging, swimming or cycling. This can be a dance class if you like – anything will do, from salsa to line-dancing to belly-dancing. When you are feeling better, you may like to try playing a competitive sport – like tennis, football, cricket, squash or badminton – they all count as aerobic exercise. Try to alternate your choices as much as possible, so you get a good mix throughout the programme.

Where you see this icon **P**, you should choose a Pilates or yoga session, a resistance/weight-training exercise session, or something similar. If you do a class on these days, that's perfect.

If you are doing weight training, you need to pay attention to the U and L symbols – they do not apply to any other exercises. They are there to remind you to exercise both your stomach and upper body (U) and your stomach and lower body (L) , so that you work all parts of your body over the period.

The time you spend exercising is short to begin with and gradually increases as the programme progresses. However, if you participate in an exercise class, do try to complete it – don't walk out after the allotted time in your programme! If you think about it, a lot of time during an organised class is taken up with getting ready, talking to and watching the instructor as you learn a new exercise and waiting whilst the instructor helps individuals. When you work out at home, it is much more concentrated.

Week	Monday	Tuesday	Wednesday	Thursday	Friday	Saturday	Sunday
3		**A** 15 mins		**P** (U) 20 mins		**A** 20 mins	
4	**P** (L) 20 mins		**A** 15 mins		**A** 20 mins		
5		**A** 20 mins		**P** (U) 20 mins		**P** (L) 25 mins	
6	**A** 15 mins		**A** 25 mins		**P** (U) 20 mins		
7	**A** 20 mins		**A** 20 mins		**A** 20 mins		**P** (L) 20 mins
8	**A** 25 mins				**P** (U) 20 mins		**A** 20 mins
9	**P** (L) 20 mins		**A** 20 mins		**A** 25 mins		**A** 25 mins
10		**A** 25 mins		**P** (U) 20 mins		**A** 25 mins	

The maintenance stage

Once you have completed this 10-week programme, you should feel so comfortable with your routine that you can progress it yourself.

The first thing to do is add five minutes to each session and work through the 10-week programme again. You can keep doing this until your sessions reach one hour – which is quite long enough! If you still feel you want to go further, you can then add one more session per week, keeping the sessions spaced out, and then work through the 10-week programme again.

Don't go too far: you should always have at least one or two days off per week and there is no need to exercise for over an hour at a time to gain physical and mental benefits.

chapter twelve

Stocking up for Easy Eating

S hopping for food – and cooking it – can feel like insurmountable obstacles when you are depressed, but it is important that you maintain a balanced diet. One way to make these chores easier is to keep your kitchen well-stocked with everyday food items so that you can put together a nourishing snack or meal whenever you want it, without having to go to the effort of going to the shops.

The lists on the following pages are intended purely as a guide for you to make your own selection, but I would recommend that you keep a good range of the cans and packets as these have a long shelf life. If you have a freezer, you will be able to store many more fresh foods too. I have included a full list of fresh fruit and vegetables, meat and dairy products that will be particularly useful, but don't buy too many at once, or you will waste them.

Ready meals provide an excellent stand-by for those days when you don't feel like cooking. Choose those that include vegetables and any necessary accompaniments, such as rice and follow the tips on making ready meals healthy on page 28.

If you aren't well enough to go shopping yourself, either order over the internet or ask a friend or relative to do it for you.

Note: In the lists I have suggested low-fat and low-sugar varieties where appropriate. As I have already explained, too much sugar and fat will only increase your depression, but if you really can't do without butter and sweet things, try to cut down the amount you eat of these and substitute other foods wherever possible.

Canned foods

You can make a complete meal from canned items, so choose your favourites and keep a good range in stock.

- Apricots in natural juice
- Asparagus, cut
- Baked beans in tomato sauce
- Button mushrooms
- Chicken in white sauce
- Creamed rice pudding, preferably low-fat
- Macaroni cheese
- Minced (ground) beef with onion
- Peas and baby carrots
- Pilchards in tomato sauce
- Pineapple in natural juice
- Prunes in natural juice, or breakfast compôte
- Red kidney beans
- Salmon
- Sardines
- Soups – cream of tomato, chunky meat and/or vegetable, lentil or bean
- Sweetcorn
- Tomatoes
- Tuna
- Vegetable ravioli in tomato sauce

Packets

These items last well, as long as you remember to keep them in a cool store cupboard. Close open packets or store them in airtight containers.

- Breakfast cereals, preferably wholegrain varieties
- Chinese egg noodles
- Chocolate, plain (semi-sweet), good-quality, with at least 70 per cent cocoa solids, such as Green and Black's or one of the Belgian brands
- Coconut, shredded (desiccated)
- Couscous
- Digestive biscuits (graham crackers)
- Dried fruit and nut cereal bars, preferably with low added sugar
- Dried fruits – dates, apricots, prunes, peaches, raisins, sultanas (golden raisins), figs, blueberries, cranberries
- Instant hot oat cereal
- Instant mashed potato
- Microwave or quick-cook long-grain rice
- Mushroom risotto
- Nuts – walnuts, pine nuts, almonds, brazils, cashews, peanuts
- Oatcakes
- Pasta, quick-cook
- Porridge oats
- Rye or other wholegrain crispbreads or crackers
- Savoury rice
- Seeds – pumpkin, sunflower, sesame
- Stuffed dried tortellini with spinach and ricotta
- Wheatgerm

Sundries

This section contains all the items you need to add interest and flavour to your meals.

- Dried herbs – oregano, basil, parsley, mixed herbs
- French dressing
- Garlic purée (paste)
- Honey, clear
- Lemon juice, bottled
- Mango chutney and/or sweet pickle
- Marmalade, preferably reduced-sugar
- Marmite or other yeast extract
- Mayonnaise, preferably low-fat
- Mustard
- Oils – olive and sunflower
- Pasta stir-in sauces
- Peanut butter
- Salt and pepper
- Soy sauce
- Spices – ground cinnamon and cumin, curry powder or paste, chilli powder
- Tabasco or hot chilli sauce
- Tomato ketchup (catsup)
- Tomato purée (paste)
- Vinegars – balsamic, red and white wine
- Worcestershire sauce

Drinks

- Bedtime drinks – Ovaltine, Horlicks, drinking chocolate
- Coffee and tea, decaffeinated
- Pure fruit juices – orange, apple, tomato

Frozen foods

These foods can be bought ready-frozen but you can also store many other fresh foods in your freezer, as long as you wrap and seal them well. Check the labels for suitability.

- Char-grilled chicken fillets
- Chopped spinach
- Cooked prawns (shrimp)
- Ice cream, preferably low-fat
- Mixed vegetables
- Peas
- Raspberries
- Rosti
- Salmon fillets

Bakery items

Many of these can also be stored in a freezer. You can take out individual items as you need them and thaw them in your microwave or under the grill (broiler).

- Bagels
- Bread, preferably multigrain or wholemeal
- Bread rolls, wholegrain
- Currant buns/tea cakes
- Flour tortillas
- Naans (plain)
- Pittas, preferably wholemeal or sesame seed

Fresh meat, dairy products, etc.

Do not buy too many fresh foods at once and remember to keep an eye on their 'best by' dates.

- Bacon

- Butter or, preferably, a low-fat spread, suitable for cooking and spreading

- Cheeses – white soft cheese, such as ricotta or cottage; fresh Mozzarella, feta and goats' cheese; hard cheeses, such as Cheddar and Parmesan (buy ready-grated where appropriate if you can't be bothered to do it yourself)

- Coleslaw

- Cooked chicken legs and breasts

- Cooked meats – beef, pork, Parma or other raw (unsmoked) cured ham

- Crème fraîche, preferably low-fat

- Eggs

- Fromage frais, plain and fruit, preferably low-fat and low-sugar

- Hummus

- Milk, preferably semi-skimmed

- Pork sausages, fresh, good quality, extra-lean

- Yoghurt, plain and fruit, preferably low-fat and low-sugar

Fresh fruit and vegetables

These are very important to your diet, but don't buy more than you can eat within two or three days. Keep a stock of your favourites and check my snack and meals plans when planning your shopping.

- Apples
- Avocados
- Baby spinach
- Bananas
- Broccoli
- Caesar salad, ready-prepared
- Carrots, ready-grated or cut into matchsticks if you like
- Celery
- Cucumber
- French beans
- Kiwi fruit
- Lettuce, ready-prepared, if you like
- Melon, preferably orange-fleshed
- Mushrooms
- Onions
- Oranges, satsumas, clementines
- Peppers (bell peppers)
- Potatoes
- Seedless grapes
- Tomatoes
- Watercress or rocket

chapter thirteen

Notes on the Recipes

 All ingredients are given in imperial, metric and American measures. Follow one set only in a recipe. American terms are given in brackets.

- The ingredients are listed in the order in which they are used in the recipe.

- All spoon measures are level: 1 tsp=5 ml; 1 tbsp=15 ml

- Eggs are medium unless otherwise stated.

- Always wash, peel, core and seed, if necessary, fresh produce before use.

- Seasoning and the use of strongly flavoured ingredients such as garlic or chillies is very much a matter of personal taste. Taste the food as you cook and adjust to suite your own palate.

- Fresh herbs are great for garnishing and adding flavour. Pots of them are available in all good supermarkets. Keep your favourite ones on the windowsill and water regularly. I use a mixture of these and dried ones in the recipes. Don't substitute dried for fresh when only fresh is called for (there is always a good reason why I've used them!)

- All can and packet sizes are approximate as they vary from brand to brand. For example, if I call for a 400 g/14 oz/large can of tomatoes and yours is a 397 g can – that's fine.

- Cooking times are approximate and should be used as a guide only. Always check food is piping hot and cooked through before serving.

- Always preheat the oven and cook on the shelf just above the centre unless otherwise stated (fan ovens do not need preheating and the positioning is not so crucial).

- I call for low-fat spread as an alternative to butter throughout the book. Choose a reduced-fat sunflower, soya or olive oil spread that is suitable for cooking as well as spreading.

- I recommend that you use skimmed or semi-skimmed milk, not full-cream, and choose low-fat varieties of cheese, cream and yoghurt, when appropriate.

A word on hygiene

Hygiene is important. Always wash your hands before preparing food and keep your kitchen clean, especially the work surfaces. If you have food left over, make sure it is completely cold before storing in the fridge in a clean, covered container. Check instructions on heating and reheating very carefully, making sure that food is piping hot (never just warm). Never refreeze anything that has thawed unless you cook it first.

chapter fourteen

Breakfasts to Brighten

Nutritionists always stress that breakfast is the most important meal of the day and when you are depressed, it is even more vital. If your body is lacking the nutrients that provide vital energy, there is no way you are going to feel on top of the world. This section gives you plenty of ideas to give you the best possible start to your day.

Always have a glass of pure fruit juice with the breakfasts that I have devised here. If you don't feel like cooking, then have a bowl of wholegrain or multigrain cereal, add some fresh or dried fruit, a handful of sunflower or pumpkin seeds and some yoghurt (plain or flavoured) or milk – that will really set you up for the day ahead. Alternatively, make one of the wake-up smoothies on pages 150 and 151. If you like tea or coffee, these should, ideally, be decaffeinated. If you can't go without a caffeine kickstart, at least don't have the real thing too strong!

Most of these recipes make meals for two people, but if you are cooking just for yourself, reduce the ingredients accordingly.

American Cheese Pancakes with Seeded Lemon Honey

You can top the pancakes with some sliced fresh strawberries or banana, a handful of blueberries or even some chopped nectarine or peach too.

SERVES 2

25 g/1 oz/¼ cup wholemeal flour
50 g/2 oz/¼ cup cottage cheese
2.5 ml/½ tsp baking powder
A good pinch of salt
1 large egg
30 ml/2 tbsp milk
A little oil for frying
30 ml/2 tbsp clear honey
Finely grated zest and juice of ½ small lemon
15 ml/1 tbsp sunflower seeds

1 Put the flour, cottage cheese, baking powder and salt in a bowl. Break in the egg and add the milk.

2 Beat well with a wooden spoon or an electric whisk until thick and well blended.

3 Heat a little oil in a large, heavy frying pan. Add about a quarter of the batter to one side of the pan and spread out to a round about 12.5 mm/4 in in diameter. Add another round of batter. Cook until golden underneath, the top is just set and bubbles are popping on the surface. Flip over and cook the other side briefly.

4 Slide on to a plate and keep warm while cooking the remaining two pancakes.

5 Meanwhile, heat the honey with the lemon zest and juice in a saucepan with the seeds.

6 Put two pancakes on each of two warm plates, spoon a little of the warm seeded honey over and serve.

Breakfast Banana, Wheatgerm and Yoghurt Muffins

There is no point in making less than this quantity – the muffins will keep in an airtight container or can be frozen, then warmed as required.

MAKES 12

2 large ripe bananas
2 large eggs, separated
150 ml/¼ pt/⅔ cup plain yoghurt
100 g/4 oz/1 cup wheatgerm
30 ml/2 tbsp sunflower oil
60 ml/4 tbsp clear honey
50 g/2 oz/⅓ cup raisins
75 g/3 oz/¾ cup wholemeal flour
5 ml/1 tsp baking powder
2.5 ml/½ tsp bicarbonate of soda (baking soda)
5 ml/1 tsp mixed (apple-pie) spice
1.5 ml/¼ tsp salt
To serve:
A little butter or low-fat spread

1 Preheat the oven to 200°C/400°F/gas 6/fan oven 180°C. Line the 12 sections of a tartlet tin (patty pan) with paper cake cases (cupcake papers).

2 Put the bananas in a bowl and mash with a fork. Add the egg yolks, yoghurt, wheatgerm, oil, honey and raisins. Mix together well.

3 Sift the flour, baking powder, bicarbonate of soda, mixed spice and salt over the surface and beat in.

4 Whisk the egg whites until stiff, then fold into the mixture with a metal spoon. Turn into the prepared tins and bake in the oven at for 20 minutes or until well risen and the centres spring back when lightly pressed.

5 Serve warm, with butter or low-fat spread, if liked.

Apple Breakfast Flummery

I keep a container of toasted oatmeal so I can make this whenever I feel like it. Try adding a few fresh blackberries when in season too.

SERVES 2

25 g/1 oz/^{1}/$_4$ cup medium oatmeal
1 eating (dessert) apple
2.5 ml/^{1}/$_2$ tsp lemon juice
250 ml/8 fl oz/1 cup plain yoghurt
15 ml/1 tbsp clear honey

1 Heat a non-stick frying pan. Add the oatmeal and toast lightly, tossing and stirring for 2–3 minutes until golden. Tip out of the pan immediately so it doesn't burn.

2 Peel, core and dice the apple. Mix with the lemon juice and toss together.

3 Mix the yoghurt with the honey, then stir in the fruit and oatmeal until evenly mixed. Spoon into glasses or bowls and serve.

Blueberry and Almond Porridge

This is equally lovely with other soft fruits, such as raspberries, strawberries or blackberries. You can use fresh, thawed frozen or soft dried fruits.

SERVES 2

75 g/3 oz/³/₄ cup rolled porridge oats
250 ml/8 fl oz/1 cup milk
175 ml/6 fl oz/³/₄ cup water
A pinch of salt
20 ml/4 tsp clear honey
25 g/1 oz/¹/₄ cup chopped toasted almonds
50 g/2 oz blueberries

1 Mix the oats with the milk, water and salt in a large saucepan.

2 Bring to the boil, reduce the heat and simmer, stirring, for 5 minutes until smooth, thick and creamy. Alternatively, cook in a bowl in the microwave, stirring every minute.

3 Stir in the honey and nuts. Spoon into bowls and top with the blueberries.

Crunchy-topped Tropical Fruit Bowl

You can prepare the fruits the night before and store them in the fridge in a covered container. If eating alone, store the remainder in the fridge for the next few mornings, but do not top with the crunch until just before serving.

SERVES 2

1 papaya or mango
1 pink grapefruit
1 small banana
1 passion fruit
15 ml/2 tbsp elderflower cordial
10 ml/2 tsp lime or lemon juice
2 crunchy almond cereal bars

1 Peel and halve the papaya, scoop out the seeds and cut the flesh into chunks. Place in a large bowl. If using a mango, cut it into two or three pieces, slicing round the stone (pit). Score the flesh in lines through to the skin in two directions, to make small cubes, then bend the skin back and cut the cubes off the skin. Place in the bowl.

2 Cut all the peel and pith from the grapefruit and cut into segments, discarding the membranes (I squeeze them over the bowl at the end to extract the last of the juice). Place in the bowl.

3 Peel and cut the banana into chunks. Add to the bowl.

4 Halve the passion fruit and scoop the seeds into the bowl.

5 Mix the elderflower cordial with the lime or lemon juice, add to the bowl and toss gently.

6 When ready to serve, roughly crush the crunchy bars with a rolling pin or a wooden spoon.

7 Spoon the fruit into bowls and sprinkle the crunchy cereal over. Serve straight away.

Mexican Scrambled Eggs

This isn't for the faint-hearted! If you don't like hot, spicy food, you could omit the chilli, but it won't have quite the same wake-up effect.

SERVES 2

A knob of butter or low-fat spread
2 spring onions (scallions), chopped
1 small red (bell) pepper, finely chopped
1 large tomato, diced
1 small green chilli, seeded and finely chopped
4 eggs
30 ml/2 tbsp crème fraîche
Salt and freshly ground black pepper
2 slices of multigrain bread, toasted
A little chopped fresh coriander (cilantro)

1   Melt the butter or spread in a non-stick saucepan. Add the spring onions and pepper and stir-fry for 3 minutes until softened slightly.

2   Add the tomato and chilli and cook, stirring, for 1 minute.

3   Beat the eggs with the crème fraîche and some salt and pepper. Add to the pan and cook over a fairly gentle heat, stirring all the time, until scrambled but still creamy.

4   Put the toast on two warm plates, top with the egg mixture and sprinkle with the coriander before serving.

Mushroom Bagels with Ham, Eggs and Cheese

Bagels are the perfect vehicles for a whole range of tasty toppings because their firm texture stops them going soggy too quickly.

SERVES 2

1 egg
2 large open-cup mushrooms
A little butter or low-fat spread
Salt and freshly ground black pepper
1 bagel, halved
4 slices of cooked ham, chopped
25 g/1 oz/¼ cup grated Cheddar cheese
10 ml/2 tsp milk
A little chopped fresh parsley

1 Boil the egg for 5 minutes, then plunge into cold water. Drain and remove the shell.

2 Meanwhile, peel the mushrooms. Spread on both sides with a little butter or low-fat spread and a sprinkling of salt and pepper, and place on foil on the grill (broiler) rack, gill-sides down. Grill (broil) for 3 minutes, then turn over. Add the bagel halves to the grill and cook for a further 2 minutes, cut sides down, then turn the bagels over and cook for a further 1 minute.

3 Meanwhile, chop the boiled egg and mix with the ham, grated cheese and milk.

4 Put the mushrooms on the bagels, then pile the egg mixture on top, spreading out to cover the bagels. Grill for 2 minutes until the cheese is turning lightly golden and bubbling.

5 Transfer the bagels to warm plates and scatter a little chopped parsley over.

Wake-up Fruit Smoothie

This is the perfect start for anyone who can't be bothered to eat! If this is too fiddly, use two bananas and omit the other fruits, or experiment with any other combination you like. Always use a banana as a base as it gives the lovely thick, smooth texture to the finished smoothie – as well as packing it with goodness.

SERVES I

1 large banana
1 eating (dessert) apple, peeled, cored and sliced
1 nectarine, peach or wedge of melon, stone (pit) or seeds removed,
cut into pieces
5 ml/1 tsp clear honey
30 ml/2 tbsp wheatgerm
200 ml/7 fl oz/scant 1 cup milk

1   Put all the ingredients in a blender or food processor and run the machine until thick and smooth.

2   Pour into a very large glass and serve.

Wake-up Savoury Smoothie

This is a far more sophisticated than the usual fruit smoothies. You can experiment with other canned or fresh cooked vegetables or try using mixed vegetable (V8) juice instead of tomato.

SERVES I

1 × 295 g/10¹/₂ oz/medium can of carrots in water
¹/₂ small avocado, peeled, stoned (pitted) and cut into chunks
¹/₂ small red (bell) pepper, cut into rough chunks
300 ml/¹/₂ pt/1¹/₄ cups tomato juice
1.5 ml/¹/₄ tsp celery or onion salt
15 ml/1 tbsp wheatgerm
Freshly ground black pepper
75 ml/5 tbsp water
Ice cubes (optional) and good splash of Worcestershire
and/or Tabasco sauce

1 Put the carrots with their water in a blender or food processor. Add all the remaining ingredients except the sauces and run the machine until the mixture is smooth.

2 Pour into a large glass and add ice cubes, if liked, and Worcestershire and/or Tabasco to taste.

chapter fifteen

Light and Luscious Lunches or Suppers

hese light meals are designed to make you feel on top of the world. But if you don't want to be bothered to cook or are eating out for any reason, you can still make sure you have a balanced meal with all the nutrients you need. Avoid junk food, such as pies, burgers and anything with chips (fries). Instead go for wholemeal or granary bread sandwiches or wraps with fish, chicken or cheese and salad fillings. For hot snacks, choose good-quality soups made with pulses (dried peas, beans or lentils), vegetables, rice or other grains, chicken, meat or fish. Another tasty option is a jacket-baked potato, with beans, cheese, seafood or vegetable topping.

Quick Broccoli Cheese

You could make this with cauliflower if you prefer. It really is full of flavour and goodness and much quicker to make than one with a 'proper' cheese sauce.

SERVES 2

1 head of broccoli (about 225 g/8 oz), separated into florets
50g/2 oz/^{1}/$_2$ cup grated Cheddar cheese (about 2 handfuls)
^{1}/$_2$ × 200 g/7 oz carton of crème fraîche
2.5 ml/^{1}/$_2$ tsp made English mustard
A pinch of dried mixed herbs
2 tomatoes, quartered, or 8 cherry tomatoes
Salt and freshly ground black pepper
To serve:
Wholemeal bread with a little butter or low-fat spread

1 Cook the broccoli in boiling, lightly salted water for about 4 minutes until just tender but not soft. Drain well.

2 Add the cheese, crème fraîche, mustard and mixed herbs to the pan and heat gently, stirring until the cheese melts. Allow to bubble for 2 minutes to thicken slightly.

3 Return the broccoli to the pan with the tomatoes and heat, stirring gently and folding over in the sauce, until everything is hot through but the tomatoes still have some shape.

4 Spoon into bowls and serve with wholemeal bread with a little butter or low-fat spread.

Spiced Chick Pea Soup with Raisins

This has a lovely exotic flavour. If you aren't keen on the idea of sweet raisins in it, substitute pine nuts.

SERVES 2–4

15 ml/1 tbsp olive oil
1 onion, chopped
5 ml/1 tsp garlic purée (paste)
5 ml/1 tsp ground cumin
2.5 ml/¹/₂ tsp ground cinnamon
250 ml/8 fl oz/1 cup passata
600 ml/1 pt /2¹/₂ cups vegetable stock, made with 1 stock cube
30 ml/2 tbsp tomato purée (paste)
1 × 425 g/15 oz/large can of chick peas (garbanzos), drained
75 ml/5 tbsp instant potato flakes
50 g/2 oz/¹/₃ cup raisins
2.5 ml/¹/₂ tsp dried oregano
1 bay leaf
2.5 ml/¹/₂ tsp clear honey
Salt and freshly ground black pepper
To serve:
Wholemeal pitta breads

1 Heat the oil in a large saucepan and add the onion. Cook, stirring, for 2 minutes.

2 Stir in the spices, then all the remaining ingredients. Bring to the boil, reduce the heat, part-cover and simmer for 10 minutes.

3 Discard the bay leaf, then taste and re-season if necessary.

4 Serve with warm wholemeal pittas.

Quick Cheese and Vegetable Soup

This is one of my favourite soups – heartwarming, tasty and very quick to make. You could sprinkle some crisply cooked crumbled bacon over the surface for added texture and flavour.

SERVES 2–4

1 × 300 g/11 oz/medium can of diced mixed vegetables
450 ml/³/₄ pt/2 cups vegetable stock, made with 1 stock cube
300 ml/¹/₂ pt/1¹/₄ cups milk
30 ml/2 tbsp cornflour (cornstarch)
100 g/4 oz/1 cup grated Cheddar cheese
2.5 ml/¹/₂ tsp celery salt
5 ml/1 tsp dried chives
Freshly ground black pepper
To serve:
Granary rolls

1   Empty the vegetables with their liquid into a saucepan with the stock.

2   Blend the milk and cornflour together, then add to the pan. Bring to the boil, stirring, and cook for 1 minute.

3   Add the cheese, celery salt and chives and cook, stirring, for 1 minute until the cheese has melted. Season with pepper.

4   Serve hot with granary rolls.

Curried Lentil and Tomato Soup

Warming, tasty and very nutritious, this is the ideal soup for a cold day.
If you have any other root vegetables, such as a parsnip or piece of swede,
pop that in too!

SERVES 2–4

10 ml/2 tsp olive oil
1 onion, roughly chopped
2 carrots, roughly chopped
10 ml/2 tsp curry paste
100 g/4 oz/²/₃ cup red lentils
600 ml/1 pt/2¹/₂ cups chicken or vegetable stock,
made with 1 stock cube
1 × 400 g/14 oz/large can of chopped tomatoes
30 ml/2 tbsp tomato purée (paste)
5 ml/1 tsp clear honey
Salt and freshly ground black pepper
30 ml/2 tbsp desiccated (shredded) coconut, for garnishing
To serve:
Warm naan breads

1 Heat the oil in a saucepan over a moderate heat. Add the onion and carrots and fry, stirring, for 2 minutes, until softened but not browned. Stir in the curry paste.

2 Add all the remaining ingredients. Bring to the boil, reduce the heat, part-cover and simmer for about 30 minutes until the lentils and carrots are completely soft. Liquidise in a blender or food processor. Return to the pan and heat through.

3 Taste the soup and re-season, if necessary. Ladle into warm bowls and garnish each with a little desiccated coconut.

4 Serve with warm naan breads.

Cheese and Rocket Bagels

This is a lovely way of including a good portion of greens without having to munch your way through them! Use watercress if you prefer.

SERVES 2 OR 4

1 × 50 g/2 oz packet of rocket
100 g/4 oz/1 cup of grated Cheddar cheese (about 4 handfuls)
60 ml/4 tbsp mayonnaise
A good grinding of black pepper
2 bagels
A little butter or low-fat spread
20 ml/4 tsp tomato purée (paste)
Salt and freshly ground black pepper

1 Put the rocket in a bowl and snip into small pieces with scissors.

2 Mix in the cheese and mayonnaise, then season well with pepper.

3 Meanwhile, split the bagels and toast on both sides under the grill (broiler).

4 Spread with a little butter or low-fat spread, then the tomato purée.

5 Pile the cheese mixture on top and spread out slightly, then grill (broil) for 2 minutes until the cheese bubbles and turns lightly golden on top.

Spinach, Pancetta and Ricotta Frittata

This is a classy Italian omelette. Experiment with goats' cheese instead of ricotta and mushrooms instead of the pancetta – just sauté them in a knob of butter or low-fat spread before adding the egg mixture.

SERVES 2

100 g/4 oz frozen leaf spinach, thawed
4 eggs
50 g/2 oz/¼ cup ricotta cheese
Salt and freshly ground black pepper
5 ml/1 tsp olive oil
50 g/2 oz diced pancetta
To serve:
Wholemeal toast and butter or low-fat spread

1 Squeeze the thawed spinach to remove as much moisture as possible, then snip into small pieces with scissors.

2 Whisk the eggs together with the cheese and a little salt and pepper.

3 Heat the oil in a large non-stick frying pan, add the pancetta and cook until golden, stirring all the time.

4 Scatter the spinach in the pan, then pour in the egg and cheese mixture. Cook, lifting and stirring, until the mixture is golden brown underneath and almost set.

5 Meanwhile, preheat the grill (broiler). Put the pan under the grill and cook until the top is golden.

6 Cut in half and serve with slices of wholemeal toast, with a little butter or low-fat spread.

Garlic, Mozzarella, Tomato and Olive Bread

This is a really moreish way to serve garlic bread. Just buy a ready-to-bake loaf – a cheap 'economy' one is ideal for this as the recipe adds so many good things.

SERVES 2–4

1 ready-to-bake garlic baguette
1 × 125 g/4¹/₂ oz fresh Mozzarella cheese, drained and sliced
2 tomatoes, sliced
A handful of sliced black or green olives
A few chopped fresh or a pinch of dried basil
To serve:
A green salad

1 Preheat the oven to 200°C/400°F/gas 6/fan oven 180°C.

2 Unwrap the bread and put it on a baking (cookie) sheet.

3 Push a slice of cheese and tomato into each cut. Add a few sliced olives. Sprinkle with the basil.

4 Bake in the oven for about 10 minutes until golden and the cheese had melted.

5 Cut into portions and serve hot with a green salad.

Cracked Wheat Salad with Pumpkin Seeds, Pear and Feta Cheese

This is a delicious sweet and salty salad. If you like hot, spicy food, add a chopped fresh chilli or a few dried chilli flakes.

SERVES 2

100 g/4 oz/³/₄ cup bulgar (cracked wheat)
300 ml/¹/₂ pt/1¹/₄ cups boiling water
1 small green (bell) pepper, diced
1 ripe pear, peeled, cored and sliced
30 ml/2 tbsp pumpkin seeds
2 spring onions (scallions), trimmed and chopped
75 g/3 oz/¹/₃ cup feta cheese, cubed
A small handful of black olives
4 cherry tomatoes, halved
30 ml/2 tbsp olive oil
10 ml/2 tsp lemon juice
10 ml/2 tsp dried mint
Salt and freshly ground black pepper

1 Put the bulgar saucepan. Add the boiling water. Stir, bring back to the boil and simmer for 10–15 minutes until all the water is absorbed and the bulgar is tender.

2 Stir in all the remaining ingredients and serve straight away. Alternatively, leave until cold, then chill before serving.

Griddled Tortilla Wedges with Cheese and Ham

This is based on the famous Mexican quesadillas. They make a great snack any time of day. You can have plain cheese or add other fillings, such as chopped chicken and some chilli salsa instead of the ham, for a change.

SERVES 2

**2 flour tortillas
4 slices of ham
8 thin slices of Cheddar cheese
A few drops of Tabasco sauce (optional)**
To serve:
A small mixed salad

1 Put one tortilla on a board and cover with the ham, then the cheese, in an even layer. Add drops over Tabasco over the surface, if liked.

2 Top with the other tortilla and press down well.

3 Heat a large heavy-based frying pan. Turn down the heat to moderate. Add the tortilla 'sandwich' and heat, pressing down on top with a fish slice until the tortilla is golden underneath.

4 Carefully turn the 'sandwich' over and cook, pressing down all the time, until golden underneath and the cheese has melted. Cut into wedges and serve with a mixed salad.

chapter sixteen

Main Meals to Make You Smile

T hese recipes are all a bit unusual – which makes mealtimes more interesting – but very easy to make and absolutely wonderful to eat. They are also packed with all the nourishment you need to boost your spirits and your energy levels.

If you don't want to cook, or are eating out, choose a pasta or rice dish with salad or grilled meat, fish or poultry, with fresh vegetables or salad, or main meal salads, such as Caesar Salad, Salade Niçoise, etc. Avoid anything deep-fried as well as dishes smothered in very rich fatty sauces – they will make you feel slow and sluggish and are hard to digest, especially late at night.

Gnocchi, Tuna and Spring Green Bake

Try this with some diced blue cheese or ham instead of the tuna for other great flavour combinations.

SERVES 2–4

1 × 350 g/12 oz packet of gnocchi
1 head of spring (collard) greens, finely shredded,
discarding the thick central stump
1 × 185 g/6¹/₂ oz/small can of tuna, drained
1 × 295 g/10¹/₂ oz/medium can of condensed mushroom soup
50 g/2 oz/¹/₂ cup grated Cheddar cheese
To serve:
A tomato salad

1 Cook the gnocchi and the greens together in boiling, lightly salted water for 3 minutes. Preheat the oven to 200°C/400°F/gas 6/fan oven 180°C.

2 Drain both thoroughly and turn into a shallow baking dish.

3 Scatter the tuna over.

4 Spoon the soup over, then sprinkle with the cheese.

5 Bake in the oven for about 25 minutes until golden and bubbling.

6 Serve hot with a tomato salad.

Chicken in a Pan with Cider, Beans, Potatoes and Apples

This is a quick, all-in-one dish that's great for any occasion. You can add some sliced carrots at the same time as the potatoes for extra goodness.

SERVES 2

A knob of butter or low-fat spread
2 skinless chicken breasts
225 g/8 oz baby potatoes, scrubbed
120 ml/4 fl oz/¹/₂ cup medium cider
120 ml/4 fl oz/¹/₂ cup chicken stock, made with ¹/₂ stock cube
100 g/4 oz French (green) beans, topped, tailed
and cut into short lengths
1 eating (dessert) apple, cored and sliced, peel left on
2.5 ml/¹/₂ tsp dried mixed herbs
Salt and freshly ground black pepper
75 ml/5 tbsp crème fraîche

1   Heat the butter or spread in a large shallow pan. Add the chicken and brown on all sides.

2   Add the potatoes, cider and stock. Bring to the boil, cover, turn down the heat and simmer for 15 minutes.

3   Add the beans, apple, herbs and a little seasoning. Re-cover and simmer for a further 5 minutes until the chicken and vegetables are tender.

4   Lift the chicken and vegetables out of the pan with a draining spoon and transfer to warm plates.

5   Boil the juices rapidly for a minute or two to reduce and thicken slightly (this may not be necessary). Stir in the crème fraîche and heat through. Taste and re-season.

6   Spoon over the chicken and vegetables and serve straight away.

Spicy Coconut Prawns with Mushrooms and Courgettes on Brown Rice

This fabulous dish is so easy to make, it will soon be a favourite. It is full of nutritious things but packed with exotic flavours too. Remember, Thai curries are much runnier than Indian ones.

SERVES 2

100 g/4 oz/½ cup brown rice
½ × 400 ml/14 oz/large can of coconut milk
15 ml/1 tbsp Thai red curry paste
75 ml/5 tbsp fish stock, made with ½ stock cube
4 spring onions (scallions)
1 courgette (zucchini), cut into thick slices
50 g/2 oz baby button mushrooms, left whole
200 g/7 oz frozen raw shelled large prawns (jumbo shrimp), thawed
5–10 ml/1–2 tsp lemon or lime juice
Salt and freshly ground black pepper
1 tomato, cut into 8 pieces

1   Cook the rice in plenty of boiling, lightly salted water for about 30 minutes until tender. Drain.

2   Meanwhile, mix the coconut milk with the curry paste and stock in a saucepan. Bring to the boil, stirring.

3   Chop the spring onions, reserving a few of the dark green tops for garnish. Add to the pan with the courgettes and mushrooms and simmer for 6–8 minutes until tender.

4   Add the prawns, lemon juice and a little salt and pepper and cook gently for 3 minutes until the prawns are pink. Add the tomatoes and cook for 1 minute more.

5   Spoon the rice into warm bowls and top with the prawn mixture.

6   Sprinkle with the reserved chopped spring onion greens and serve.

Teriyaki Salmon
with Vegetable Sesame Noodles

Teriyaki marinade is easy to use – just add it straight from the bottle, nothing extra is needed to give a fabulous flavour. You can make this recipe with chicken breasts too, but you'll need to cook them for about 15 minutes, turning once or twice.

SERVES 2

2 salmon steaks
60 ml/4 tbsp teriyaki sauce
2 slabs of Chinese egg noodles
15 ml/1 tbsp sunflower oil
$^1/_2$ × 500 g/18 oz packet of frozen stir-fry vegetables
15 ml/1 tbsp sesame seeds
A few drops of soy sauce

1 Put the salmon steaks in a shallow dish and spoon the teriyaki sauce over. Turn the fish pieces over to coat completely and leave to marinate for 30 minutes.

2 Soak the noodles in boiling water for 5 minutes, then drain.

3 Heat the oil in a large frying pan or wok and stir-fry the vegetables for 5 minutes. Add the sesame seeds and fry for a further 2 minutes.

4 Meanwhile, heat the grill (broiler). Lift the fish out of the marinade and transfer to foil on the grill rack. Grill (broil) for 6 minutes.

5 Throw the noodles into the stir-fried vegetables and toss well, adding any remaining marinade from the fish.

6 Pile on to plates and top with the salmon steaks. Sprinkle a few drops of soy sauce round the edges of the plates.

Seafood Pies

Filo pastry contains very little fat so is much better for you than other types. The other lovely thing about these pies is that the pastry is completely separate, so it doesn't go soggy!

SERVES 2

1 × 225 g/8 oz/small can of chopped tomatoes
75 ml/5 tbsp apple juice
5 ml/1 tsp dried onion granules
1 rectangular frozen cod steak, cut into cubes
200 g/7 oz frozen seafood cocktail
10 ml/2 tsp cornflour (cornstarch)
2.5 ml/½ tsp garlic purée (paste)
15 ml/1 tbsp tomato purée
A pinch of dried basil
2.5 ml/½ tsp clear honey
Salt and freshly ground black pepper
2 sheets of filo pastry (paste), thawed if frozen
A little sunflower oil
75 ml/5 tbsp crème fraîche
To serve:
New potatoes, broccoli and peas

1 Put the tomatoes and apple juice in a saucepan with the onion granules. Bring to the boil and boil for 5 minutes until very thick, stirring occasionally.

2 Mix the cod and seafood with the cornflour. Stir into the tomato mixture with the garlic and tomato purées, basil and honey, and season lightly with salt and pepper.

3 Bring back to the boil, reduce the heat and simmer for 5 minutes, stirring gently occasionally.

4 Meanwhile, preheat the oven to 190°C/375°F/gas 5/fan oven 170°C. Brush the sheets of pastry with a little oil and crumple them up gently as if they were sheets of paper. Place on a lightly oiled baking (cookie) sheet. Bake for about 5 minutes until golden.

5 Stir the crème fraîche into the seafood mixture. Do not allow to boil again.

6 Spoon the fish mixture on to plates and top each with a crumpled filo sheet. Serve with new potatoes, broccoli and peas.

Quick Cassoulet

A rustic dish, full of flavour and goodness but so easy to make. You can use spicy sausages if you like them – but make sure they have a very high meat content.

SERVES 2

2 thick extra-lean meaty pork sausages, cut into chunks
2 rashers (slices) of back bacon, cut into pieces
1 skinless chicken breast, cut into chunks
1 × 425 g/15 oz/large can of haricot (navy) beans, drained
10 ml/2 tsp clear honey
120 ml/4 fl oz/¹/₂ cup chicken stock, made with 1 stock cube
2.5 ml/¹/₂ tsp garlic purée (paste)
10 ml/2 tsp tomato purée
1.5 ml/¹/₄ tsp dried mixed herbs
Salt and freshly ground black pepper
1 Weetabix, crumbled
To serve:
A green salad

1 Preheat the oven to 180°C/350°F/gas 4/fan oven 160°C. In a flameproof casserole (Dutch oven), quickly dry-fry the sausages and bacon until the fat and juices run. Add the chicken and fry for 1 further minute, stirring.

2 Add all the remaining ingredients, except the Weetabix, seasoning lightly with salt and pepper. Stir well. Bring to the boil, cover and bake in the oven for 30 minutes.

3 Remove the lid and sprinkle the top with the crushed Weetabix. Return to the oven, uncovered, and cook for a further 15 minutes.

4 Serve with a green salad.

Beef, Potato and Mixed Vegetable Bake

I created this dish many years ago but without the additional vegetables. This version gives you a complete meal in one pot – the perfect, simple supper solution.

SERVES 2

2 medium potatoes
1 × 410 g/14¹/₂ oz/large can of stewed steak in gravy
1 × 410 g/14¹/₂ oz/large can of Chinese mixed vegetables, drained
6 cup mushrooms, sliced
1 × 170 g/6 oz/small can of condensed cream of mushroom soup
30 ml/2 tbsp water

1 Slice the potatoes and boil in lightly salted water for 3 minutes until almost tender. Drain.

2 Preheat the oven to 190°C/375°F/gas 5/fan oven 170°C. Put the beef and mixed vegetables in a pie dish and mix well. Scatter the mushrooms over.

3 Spoon half the soup over and spread out.

4 Layer the sliced potatoes over the surface, overlapping as necessary.

5 Mix the rest of the soup with the water and spread over the surface of the potatoes. Bake in the oven for about 50 minutes until golden on top and piping hot.

Speciality Pizza

*I always buy the stone-baked Italian pizzas as they taste much more
authentic and have less fat in them. If you are vegetarian, omit the ham.*

SERVES 2

1 large Marguerita (cheese and tomato) pizza
4 button mushrooms, sliced
1 slice of Parma or cooked ham, diced
2 tomatoes, sliced
1 small fresh Mozzarella cheese, drained and thinly sliced
2 black olives
10 ml/2 tsp olive oil
A few fresh basil leaves, torn
A handful of fresh rocket
To serve:
A green salad and some Extra-good Garlic Bread (see page 183)

1 Unwrap the pizza and place on a baking (cookie) sheet. Preheat the
   oven according to the packet directions.

2 Scatter the mushrooms and ham over the pizza, then top with the
   tomatoes, the slices of cheese and the olives.

3 Bake in the oven for about 20 minutes or until the edge is crisp
   and golden and the cheese has melted and is bubbling.

4 Scatter the basil over, then top with the rocket.

5 Serve hot with a green salad and some Extra-good Garlic Bread.

Chicken Wrapped in Parma Ham with Pesto Spaghetti

Spaghetti has a surprising amount of goodness in it and this is a very simple meal to prepare. Make sure you have some salad with it too for a completely balanced meal. If you like wholemeal spaghetti, that's even better for you than the plain white variety.

SERVES 2

2 skinless chicken breasts
2 thin slices of Parma or other unsmoked dry-cured ham
15 ml/1 tbsp pine nuts
15 ml/1 tbsp olive oil
Salt and freshly ground black pepper
175 g/6 oz spaghetti
30 ml/2 tbsp ready-made pesto sauce
Grated Parmesan cheese, for garnishing
To serve:
A rocket and tomato salad

1 Wrap each chicken breast in a slice of Parma ham. Season lightly.

2 Heat a large frying pan (skillet), add the pine nuts and cook, stirring and turning, until the pine nuts are golden. Tip out of the pan on to a cold plate to prevent further cooking.

3 Add the oil to the pan and heat. Add the chicken and fry quickly on all sides to brown, then turn down the heat, cover with a lid or foil and cook gently for 15 minutes.

4 Meanwhile, cook the spaghetti in plenty of boiling, lightly salted water for 10 minutes or until just tender but still with some 'bite'. Drain and return to the pan. Add the pesto and toss gently over a low heat until thoroughly coated.

5 Pile the spaghetti on to warm plates. Top with the chicken and spoon any oil and juices from the pan over. Scatter the pine nuts over.

6 Dust with Parmesan and serve with a large rocket and tomato salad.

Moroccan-style Chicken
with Chick Pea and Date Couscous

You can use a can of apricots instead of peaches and lamb neck fillets instead of the chicken, if you prefer.

SERVES 2

100 g/4 oz/³/₄ cup couscous
450 ml/³/₄ pt/2 cups boiling chicken or vegetable stock,
made with 1 stock cube
20 ml/4 tsp tomato purée (paste)
5 ml/1 tsp ground cumin
25 g/1 oz/3 tbsp chopped dried dates
1 × 425 g/15 oz/large can of chick peas (garbanzos), drained
15 ml/1 tbsp olive oil
1 small onion, chopped
1 small green (bell) pepper, diced
2 skinless chicken breasts, cut into dice
2.5 ml/¹/₂ tsp garlic purée
2.5 ml/¹/₂ tsp ground cinnamon
¹/₂ × 300 ml/11 oz/medium can of sliced peaches in natural juice,
diced
Salt and freshly ground black pepper
A little chopped fresh parsley or coriander (cilantro), for garnishing
To serve:
A green salad

1 Put the couscous in a saucepan. Pour over 300 ml/¹/₂ pt/1¹/₄ cups of the stock, 10 ml/2 tsp of the tomato purée, 2.5 ml/¹/₂ tsp of the cumin, the dates and chick peas and leave to stand while you make the sauce.

2 Heat the oil in a saucepan. Add the onion and pepper and cook, stirring, for 2 minutes. Add the chicken and stir gently for 1 minute.

3 Stir in the remaining stock and tomato purée and all the remaining ingredients except the cornflour and water. Bring to the boil, reduce the heat and simmer gently for 10 minutes, stirring occasionally. Taste and re-season if necessary.

4 When the sauce is simmering, put the bowl of couscous over the saucepan and cover with a lid.

5 When cooked, remove the bowl of couscous. Blend the cornflour with the water and stir into the chicken. Bring back to the boil and cook, stirring, for 1 minute until thickened. Taste and re-season, if necessary.

6 Spoon the couscous into bowls and place the chicken on top. Garnish with parsley or coriander and serve with a green salad.

Ratatouille-stuffed Cabbage Leaves with Pine Nuts

This is an old favourite of mine and is a lovely way to use the outer leaves from a cabbage.

SERVES 2–4

8 large dark-green savoy cabbage leaves
1 × 425 g/15 oz/large can of ratatouille
60 ml/4 tbsp uncooked long-grain rice
30 ml/2 tbsp pine nuts
450 ml/³/₄ pt/2 cups vegetable stock, made with 1 stock cube
Salt and freshly ground black pepper
1.5 ml/¹/₄ tsp dried basil
100 g/4 oz/1 cup grated Cheddar cheese
To serve:
Crusty bread

1 Cut the thick central stalk off the cabbage leaves and discard. Drop the leaves into a pan of boiling water and cook for 3 minutes. Drain and rinse with cold water, then drain again.

2 Mix together the ratatouille, rice and pine nuts and put the mixture in the centres of the cabbage leaves. Fold in the sides, then roll up and place in a flameproof casserole dish (Dutch oven).

3 Pour the stock over. Season and sprinkle with the dried basil. Bring to the boil, turn down the heat, cover and simmer very gently for 30 minutes until the cabbage and rice are tender and the sauce is thick.

4 Transfer to warm plates, sprinkle with cheese and serve with crusty bread.

Chicken in Hoisin Sauce
with Pak Choi and Cashew Nuts

The lovely combination of flavours and textures makes this dish great for any occasion.

SERVES 2

2 skinless chicken breasts
60 ml/4 tbsp hoisin sauce
15 ml/1 tbsp water
1 slab of Chinese egg noodles
20 ml/4 tsp sunflower oil
A handful of raw cashew nuts
2 heads of pak choi
A few drops of soy sauce

1 Make several slashes in the chicken breasts. Mix the hoisin sauce and water in a shallow dish. Add the chicken, turn over to coat completely and leave to marinate for 1–2 hours (you can cook immediately if you like, but the flavour won't be so good).

2 When ready to cook, put the noodles in a bowl. Cover with boiling water and leave to stand for 5 minutes.

3 Meanwhile, heat 10 ml/2 tsp of the oil in a frying pan. Drain the chicken from the marinade and cook for 4–5 minutes on each side until golden and cooked through. Add the remaining marinade to the pan and allow to bubble briefly.

4 Meanwhile, heat the remaining oil in a separate pan. Trim the root ends off the pak choi and cut into halves or quarters, if large. Cook in the oil for 3 minutes, turning occasionally, until just tender. Remove from the pan and keep warm.

5 Drain the noodles, add to the pan with the cashew nuts and a few drops of soy sauce and toss until hot.

6 Pile the noodles on two warm plates. Top each with a chicken breast and spoon any juices over.

7 Serve with pieces of pak choi arranged to one side of each plate.

Devilled Liver with Mushrooms on Sweet Potato Mash

I find that even people who aren't fond of liver like this. The meat is tender and succulent and the sauce rich and spicy.

SERVES 2

1 sweet potato, peeled and cut into chunks
1 potato, peeled and cut into chunks
1 head of broccoli (about 225 g/8 oz), cut into small florets
2 knobs of butter or low-fat spread
Salt and freshly ground black pepper
225 g/8 oz lamb's liver, cut into thin slices
4 mushrooms, sliced
15 ml/1 tbsp tomato ketchup (catsup)
5 ml/1 tsp mild curry paste
5–10 ml/1–2 tsp Worcestershire sauce
2.5 ml/¹/₂ tsp lemon juice
30 ml/2 tbsp water

1 Cook the sweet potato and potato together in a pan of boiling, lightly salted water for 5 minutes. Put the broccoli in a steamer or colander over the top of the pan, cover and continue to cook for about 5 minutes or until the broccoli and potatoes are tender. Remove the steamer or colander, then drain the potatoes. Add one knob of butter or low-fat spread to the potatoes, season well, then mash thoroughly.

2 Meanwhile, melt the remaining spread in a frying pan. Add the liver and mushrooms and fry quickly for 2 minutes, turn the liver over and cook for about 2 minutes just until beads of juice appear on the surface. Remove the liver from the pan and keep warm.

3 Add the remaining ingredients to the pan and bring to the boil, stirring.

4 Pile the mash on two plates. Lay the liver on top and spoon the devilled sauce over. Arrange the broccoli around the edge.

chapter seventeen

Dreamy Desserts

F ruit, low-fat yoghurt and fromage frais are all good desserts. But there are times when you want to indulge yourself. And for most people, there is no better way to make you feel better than to have a delicious sweet treat. Unfortunately, if you are feeling depressed, sugar-laden sweets and cakes will actually make you feel worse. But the good news is that this chapter is full of gorgeous – but still extremely good for you – desserts to help put you back on top of the world. When you don't feel like dessert, have a small piece of cheese and a wholegrain cracker instead.

Rhubarb and Ginger Yoghurt Syllabub

Syllabubs are traditionally made with whipped cream. This extra-light version is deliciously full of flavour but much less rich.

SERVES 2

1 egg white
10 ml/2 tsp syrup from a jar of stem ginger
250 ml/8 fl oz/1 cup rhubarb yoghurt
2 pieces of stem ginger in syrup, drained and chopped
Tiny sprigs of mint, to decorate

1 Whisk the egg white until stiff. Whisk in the ginger syrup, then gently fold in the yoghurt and about three-quarters of the ginger.

2 Turn into two wine goblets or little glass dishes and chill for 1–2 hours so the liquid begins to separate from the fluffy top. Decorate with the remaining chopped ginger and tiny sprigs of mint.

Forest Fruits Summer Pudding

This is a no-fuss version of a traditional classic. You could use all frozen raspberries or strawberries if you prefer.

SERVES 2

150 g/5 oz frozen forest fruits, thawed
15 ml/1 tbsp clear honey
3 slices of wholemeal bread, from a large loaf, crusts removed
To serve:
Crème fraîche or plain yoghurt

1 Mix the thawed fruit with the honey, adding more if it is too tart. Dip the slices of bread one at a time into the fruit, so the juices soak into one side of each slice.

2 Line two ramekin dishes (custard cups) with some of the slices, juice-coated sides out, trimming to leave no gaps.

3 Fill with the fruit, then cover with the remaining bread, cutting it to fit and making sure there are no gaps. Stand the ramekins on a plate to catch any drips. Cover each with a circle of non-stick baking parchment, then a small saucer. Place heavy weights or cans of food on top to weigh them down. Chill overnight.

4 Loosen the edges and turn out on to serving plates. Serve with crème fraîche or plain yoghurt.

Sauteéd Pineapple with Poppy Seed and Orange Sauce

*This is an unusual dessert with lots of flavour and goodness. Try it with a
small lime instead of the orange or satsuma, but omit the lemon juice
(you may need to add a trickle of honey if it is too sharp).*

SERVES 2

A knob of butter or low-fat spread
1 × 225 g/8 oz/small can of pineapple rings in natural juice, drained,
reserving the juice
15 ml/1 tbsp cornflour (cornstarch)
Finely grated zest and juice of 1 small orange, satsuma or
clementine
15 ml/1 tbsp clear honey
5 ml/1 tsp lemon juice
10 ml/2 tsp poppy seeds
To serve:
Crème fraîche

1 Melt the butter or spread in a frying pan. Add the pineapple and
fry for about 2 minutes on each side until golden at the edges.
Remove from the pan.

2 Blend the pineapple juice with the cornflour. Add to the pan with
the orange zest and juice, the honey, lemon juice and poppy seeds.
Bring to the boil and cook, stirring, for 1 minute until thickened
and clear.

3 Return the pineapple to the pan and heat through, then transfer to
warm plates.

4 Serve with a dollop of crème fraîche.

Plum and Almond Condé

Layers of creamy rice pudding enriched with ground almonds, with juicy ripe plums nestling in between – a lovely, nutritious end to your meal. You could try other fruits, like nectarines or fresh strawberries too.

SERVES 2

1 × 225 g/8 oz/small can of creamed rice pudding
25 g/1 oz/¼ cup ground almonds
4 ripe plums, stoned (pitted) and cut into chunks
15 ml/1 tbsp clear honey
15 ml/1 tbsp toasted flaked (slivered) almonds

1 Mix the rice pudding with the ground almonds and spoon half into two glasses. Top with half the chopped plums.

2 Repeat the layers, then trickle the plums with the honey and sprinkle with the flaked almonds. Chill until ready to serve.

Real Banana Splits

Everyone needs a little decadence and this is the dessert to provide it. There's just enough chocolate in the sauce to give you a high without overdoing it, but it's best to use a cream substitute, such as Elmlea Light, to keep the fat content down.

SERVES 2

25 g/1 oz/¼ cup plain (semi-sweet) chocolate with 70 per cent cocoa solids
15 g/½ oz/1 tbsp butter or low-fat spread
30 ml/2 tbsp double (heavy) cream or double cream substitute
2 bananas
4 scoops of ice cream

1 Break up the chocolate and place in a small non-stick saucepan with the butter or low-fat spread. Heat very gently, stirring, until melted.

2 Remove from the heat and beat in the cream.

3 Peel the bananas and cut into halves lengthways. Lay two halves in each of two shallow dishes, so they look like the sides of a boat, and put two scoops of ice cream in each 'boat'.

4 Reheat the sauce, if necessary. Spoon over and serve.

Raspberry and Hazelnut Yoghurt Layer

This is a bit like a trifle but with is made using yoghurt instead of custard.

SERVES 2

2 digestive biscuits (graham crackers), finely crushed
$^1\!/_2 \times$ 300 g/11 oz/medium can of raspberries in natural juice
250 ml/8 fl oz/1 cup hazelnut (filbert) yoghurt
15 ml/1 tbsp chopped toasted hazelnuts

1 Put the crushed biscuits (cookies) in the base of two small glass dishes.

2 Reserve two raspberries for decoration and dry on kitchen paper (paper towels). Spoon the remainder, and their juice, over the biscuits. Crush lightly with the back of a spoon.

3 Spoon the yoghurt over. Sprinkle with the hazelnuts and top each with a raspberry. Chill until ready to serve.

Melon with Ice Cream and Passion Fruit

The flavour of passion fruit is like no other – strong, fragrant, sweet and sharp all in one – and it adds a whole new dimension to this simple dish. You could also try scooping one into a banana smoothie (see page 150), for a tropical buzz in the mornings.

SERVES 2

1 small round orange-fleshed melon
1 passion fruit
2 scoops of lemon or vanilla ice cream

1 Cut the melon in half and scoop out the seeds.

2 Halve the passion fruit and scoop the pulp and seeds into a small dish.

3 When ready to serve, put the melon halves into two small dishes and add a scoop of ice cream in the centre. Spoon the passion fruit pulp and seeds over and serve.

Poached Figs with Lime Ricotta

When figs aren't in season, you can use dried figs in the same way. If you buy the type that are pressed in a block, rather than loose in a packet, make sure you separate them.

Serves 2

30 ml/2 tbsp undiluted blackcurrant cordial, sugar-free if possible
150 ml/¹/₄ pt/²/₃ cup red grape juice
1.5 ml/¹/₄ tsp mixed (apple-pie) spice
6 fresh figs
50 g/2 oz/¹/₄ cup ricotta cheese
Finely grated zest of ¹/₂ lime
5 ml/1 tsp sesame seeds

1 Put the blackcurrant cordial, grape juice and spice in a saucepan and bring to the boil.

2 Add the figs, turn down the heat, and simmer gently for about 20 minutes until the figs are just tender but still holding their shape.

3 Lift out of the pan with a draining spoon and put in a container. Boil the liquid rapidly until reduced by half. Pour over the figs.

4 Leave to cool, then cover and chill.

5 Mix the ricotta with the lime zest. Put the figs on plates and spoon the syrup over. Add a spoonful of the lime ricotta, sprinkle the cheese with the sesame seeds and serve.

chapter eighteen

Beautiful Bakes

....

Baking is very therapeutic if you enjoy cooking and all these recipes are packed with the good things you need to help your recovery. They are also very satisfying to make, so why not have a go?

Where fat is required in the recipes, you will see that you can use either butter or low-fat spread. Butter does give a better flavour, but too much fat in your diet will only make your depression worse, so I would really recommend that you use a low-fat alternative.

Extra-good Garlic Bread

The seeds add a lovely texture to the bread as well as giving you those few extra nutrients you need.

SERVES 2–4

1 vacuum-packed ready-to-bake garlic baguette
15 ml/1 tbsp sesame seeds
15 ml/1 tbsp sunflower seeds

1 Preheat the oven to 200°C/400°F/gas 6/fan oven 180°C.

2 Unwrap the bread and put it on a baking (cookie) sheet. Mix the seeds together. Gently open each cut in the bread and sprinkle a few seeds inside. Sprinkle the rest over the top.

3 Bake in the oven for about 15 minutes or until golden and the crust is crisp.

4 Serve hot.

Peanut Bites

These tasty, no-bake snacks are very moreish. But, as with all these snacks, try to resist eating too many in one go!

MAKES 12

1 × 200 g/7 oz packet of plain biscuits (cookies)
100 g/4 oz/¹/₂ cup butter or low-fat spread
45 ml/3 tbsp clear honey
45 ml/3 tbsp peanut butter
50 g/2 oz/¹/₂ cup raw peanuts, roughly crushed
50 g/2 oz/¹/₂ cup sunflower seeds

1 Grease a shallow 18 cm/7 in square baking tin.

2 Tip the biscuits into a bag and roughly crush with a rolling pin or bottle.

3 Melt the butter or spread with the honey and bring to the boil. Boil for 2 minutes, then stir in the peanut butter until melted. Mix in the crushed biscuits, peanuts and sunflower seeds.

4 Press the mixture into the prepared tin and chill until firm before cutting into pieces.

Easy Potato Griddle Scones

When you fancy something a little bit different, make these for breakfast, served with bacon, eggs or spread with a little butter or low-fat spread. Or try them for lunch with a hunk of cheese, some tomatoes and pickles.

MAKES 6

75 g/3 oz instant mashed potato flakes
250 ml/ 8 fl oz/1 cup boiling water
A good knob of butter or low-fat spread, plus extra for spreading
75 g/3 oz/³/₄ cup wholemeal flour
A pinch of salt
15 ml/1 tbsp baking powder

1   Put the mashed potato flakes in a bowl. Add the boiling water and butter or low-fat spread and mix well until thoroughly blended.

2   Work in the flour, salt and baking powder.

3   Pat out on a lightly floured surface to about 1 cm/¹/₂ in thick. Cut into rounds using a 7.5 cm/3 in cutter, reshaping and cutting the trimmings as necessary.

4   Heat a lightly greased, heavy-based frying pan. Add the scones (biscuits) and cook over a moderate heat for 7 minutes on each side until golden and firm. They should be moist but not soggy in the middle.

5   Serve warm, split and spread with a little butter or low-fat spread. They can be reheated briefly in a dry frying pan the next day.

Seeded Yoghurt Scones

These highly nutritious scones are best eaten the day they are made – but they are really quick to prepare. You could add a good handful of mature Cheddar cheese and an extra splash of milk to the mixture for savoury cheese scones.

MAKES ABOUT 8

100 g/4 oz/1 cup plain (all-purpose) flour
100 g/4 oz/1 cup wholemeal flour
15 ml/1 tbsp baking powder
A pinch of salt
50 g/2 oz/^{1}/$_2$ cup sunflower seeds
50 g/2 oz/^{1}/$_4$ cup butter or low-fat spread, plus extra for spreading
90 ml/6 tbsp plain yoghurt
About 60 ml/4 tbsp milk, plus extra for glazing

1 Preheat the oven to 230°C/450°F/gas 8/fan oven 210°C. Mix the flours, baking powder, salt and sunflower seeds together.

2 Add the butter or low-fat spread and rub in with your fingertips until the mixture resembles breadcrumbs.

3 Mix in the yoghurt, then enough milk to form a soft but not sticky dough.

4 Knead gently on a lightly floured surface and pat out to a round about 2 cm/³/₄ in thick. Cut into rounds using a 5 cm/2 in cutter, reshaping and cutting the trimmings as necessary.

5 Transfer to a lightly greased baking (cookie) sheet. Brush with a little milk to glaze.

6 Bake in the oven for about 12 minutes until risen and golden and the bases sound hollow when tapped. Cool slightly on a wire rack and serve warm, split and spread with a little butter or low-fat spread.

Mixed Fruit Nibblers

If you want to treat yourself, melt a 200 g/7 oz bar of good-quality plain chocolate (with at least 70 per cent cocoa solids) and spread it over the surface of the cooked bars before leaving to set. But only eat one bar a day!

MAKES 16

1 × 170 g/6 oz/small can of evaporated milk
30 ml/2 tbsp clear honey
45 ml/3 tbsp pure orange juice
50 g/2 oz/¹/₄ cup butter or low-fat spread
50 g/2 oz/¹/₄ cup light brown sugar
100 g/4 oz/²/₃ cup sultanas (golden raisins)
100 g/4 oz/²/₃ cup dried apricots, chopped
75 g/3 oz/¹/₂ cup dried cranberries
100 g/4 oz/1 cup desiccated (shredded) coconut
350 g/12 oz/3 cups rolled porridge oats

1   Grease a 28 × 18 cm/11 × 7 in rectangular shallow baking tin. Line the base with non-stick baking parchment. Preheat the oven to 180°C/350°F/gas 4/fan oven 160°C.

2   Heat the evaporated milk in a saucepan with the honey, orange juice, butter or spread and sugar. Bring to the boil and remove from the heat.

3   Stir in the remaining ingredients until thoroughly mixed.

4   Turn the mixture into the prepared tin, spread out and press down well. Bake in the oven for 30 minutes until lightly golden. Leave to cool for 10 minutes, then mark into pieces.

5   Leave until cold before removing from the tin. Store in an airtight container.

Banana Fruit and Nut Flapjacks

I know some young medical students who loved this recipe of mine so much they practically lived on them! I have added nuts to the original mix, for added nutrients, and they do provide a very well balanced snack.

MAKES 16

1 large ripe banana
75 g/3 oz/⅓ cup butter or low-fat spread
100 g/4 oz/½ cup light brown sugar
15 ml/1 tbsp clear honey
1 × 50 g/2 oz/small bag of mixed nuts and raisins, chopped
275 g/10 oz/2½ cups porridge oats

1 Grease an 18 × 28 cm/7 × 11 in shallow baking tin. Preheat the oven to 180°C/350°F/gas 4/fan oven 160°C.

2 Peel the banana and mash well in a bowl.

3 Beat in the butter or low-fat spread, sugar and honey until well blended, then stir in the mixed nuts and raisins and the oats.

4 Press the mixture into the prepared tin and bake in the oven for about 30 minutes or until golden brown.

5 Leave to cool slightly, then cut into fingers.

6 Leave until cold before removing from the tin. Store in an airtight container.

Almost Instant Carrot and Walnut Loaf

No grating, no fiddling, just a quick, all-in-one mix using ingredients you will have in your store cupboard – this really is one of the easiest cakes to make ever. It's also extremely good for you!

MAKES A 900 G/2 LB LOAF

175 g/6 oz/³/₄ cup butter or low-fat spread
175 g/6 oz/³/₄ cup light brown sugar
250 g/9 oz/2¹/₄ cups wholemeal flour
15 ml/1 tbsp baking powder
2 large eggs
1 × 300 g/11 oz/medium can of sliced carrots, drained
5 ml/1 tsp dried mixed (apple-pie) spice
50 g/2 oz/¹/₂ cup chopped walnuts
A little icing (confectioners') sugar, for dusting

1   Preheat the oven to 180°C/350°F/gas 4/fan oven 160°F. Grease a 900 g/2 lb loaf tin and line the base with non-stick baking parchment.

2   Put all the ingredients except the icing sugar in a bowl and beat with a wooden spoon until well blended (or use a hand mixer or food processor).

3   Turn into the prepared tin, level the surface and bake in the oven for about 1 hour until risen and golden.

4   Leave to cool in the tin, then turn out and dust with a little icing sugar.

Index

Recipe index

Recipe index